Promoting Self-Change from Problem Substance Use:
Practical Implications for Policy, Prevention and Treatment

Promoting Self-Change from Problem Substance Use:

Practical Implications for Policy, Prevention and Treatment

by

H. Klingemann, L. Sobell, J. Barker, J. Blomqvist,
W. Cloud, T. Ellinstad, D. Finfgeld, R. Granfield,
D. Hodgins, G. Hunt, C. Junker, F. Moggi,
S. Peele, R. Smart, M. Sobell, J. Tucker

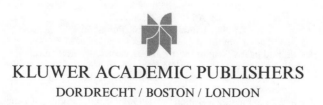

KLUWER ACADEMIC PUBLISHERS
DORDRECHT / BOSTON / LONDON

Library of Congress Cataloging-in-Publication Data is available.

ISBN (hardback) 0-7923-6771-5
ISBN (paperback) 0-7923-7088-0

Published by Kluwer Academic Publishers,
PO Box 17, 3300 AA Dordrecht, The Netherlands.

Sold and distributed in North, Central and South America
by Kluwer Academic Publishers
101 Philip Drive, Norwell, MA 02018, USA

In all other countries, sold and distributed
by Kluwer Academic Publishers, Distribution Center,
PO Box 322, 3300 AH Dordrecht, The Netherlands

Printed on acid-free paper

Printed and bound in Great Britain by MPG Books Ltd., Bodmin, Cornwall.

Dedication

This book would not have been possible without all those individuals around the world who have graciously stepped forward to '*tell their stories*' about how they changed on their own. We felt that those individuals who shared their time and experiences with us so that we could better understand the change process should also be heard. Thus, their words and feelings are sprinkled throughout this book, and it is to them that this book is dedicated.

Contents

Contents   xi

Acknowledgments

We are grateful to Dr Olaf J. Blaauw, Medical Publishing Editor, Kluwer Academic Publishers, Bio-Medical Unit, PO Box 17, 3300 AA Dordrecht, The Netherlands, and Ms. Lucienne Boujon who provided the essential secretarial backup at the Swiss Institute (secretary).

The two institutes which have shouldered a major part of the burden for this editorial project are the Center for Psychological Studies, Nova Southeastern University, Ft. Lauderdale, USA and the Swiss Institute for the Prevention of Alcohol and other Drug Problems, Lausanne, Switzerland.

Portions of this book were supported, in part, by the following funding sources: the National Institute on Alcohol Abuse and Alcoholism, USA (Grants No AA08593, R01 AA08972, K02 AA00209); the Swiss National Science Foundation (Grant 32-8626.85); and the Swiss Federal Office of Public Health (Grants 8009 and 6003).

The participation of the Swiss Institute for the Prevention of Alcohol and Drug Problems was supported by a grant from the Swiss National Science Foundation (Ref.Nr. 99.000167(8144)).

List of Authors

Harald H.J. Klingemann
University of Applied Sciences, School of Social Work, Bern, Switzerland
(Former: Swiss Institute for the Prevention of Alcohol and Drug Problems, Lausanne, Switzerland)

Linda C. Sobell
Nova Southeastern University, Center for Psychological Studies, Fort Lauderdale, Florida, USA

Judith C. Barker
Medical Anthropology Program, University of California San Francisco, San Francisco, California, USA

Jan Blomqvist
Research and Development (FoU), Social Services Administration, Stockholm, Sweden

William Cloud
University of Denver, Graduate School of Social Work, Denver, Colorado, USA

Timothy Ellinstad
Center for Psychological Studies, Nova Southeastern University, Fort Lauderdale, Florida, USA

Deborah L. Finfgeld
Sinclair School of Nursing, University of Missouri, Columbia, USA

Robert Granfield
Department of Sociology, University of Denver, Denver, USA

David Hodgins
Addiction Centre, Foothills Medical Centre, Calgary, Alberta, Canada

Geoffrey P. Hunt
Institute for Scientific Analysis, Alameda, California, USA

Christoph A. Junker
Department of Social and Preventive Medicine, University of Bern, Bern, Switzerland

Franz Moggi
Psychiatric Services, University of Bern, Bern, Switzerland

Stanton Peele
27 West Lake Blvd., Morristown, New Jersey, USA

Reginald G. Smart
Centre for Addiction and Mental Health, Toronto, Ontario, Canada

Mark B. Sobell
Nova Southeastern University, Center for Psychological Studies, Fort Lauderdale, Florida, USA

Jalie A. Tucker
Department of Health Behavior, University of Alabama, Birmingham School of Public Health, Birmingham, Alabama, USA

Introduction

The literature clearly shows that many substance abusers and problem gamblers overcome their problems without professional assistance or without using traditional self-help groups (e.g. Alcoholics Anonymous). Research into the self-change process, however, has been impeded by two things: (a) the disease concept of addiction, which has long dominated the field, is wholly inconsistent with self-change (i.e. purports that such recovery is impossible); and (b) methodological difficulties that make it hard to gain access to these 'hidden' populations. However, since the mid 1980s there has been a serious resurgence of studies examining the self-change process. As well, the topic of self-change from substance abuse has been gaining recognition and acceptance as reflected in statements like the following: (a) 'Improvement without formal treatment is not a minor or insignificant phenomenon' [1, p. 52] and (b) 'Some individuals (perhaps 20% or more) with Alcohol Dependence achieve long-term sobriety without active treatment' [2, p. 203].

In the 1990s, the study of the self-change process was approached differently. For example, several of the newer studies used both qualitative and quantitative methods to describe how individuals change using a life history/life event approach. What emerged from the methodology of these newer studies was that a cognitive appraisal process and motivation for change appeared to be associated with the self-change process. More importantly, such findings had implications for the design of new interventions. In addition, several better-designed surveys provided a basis for more precise estimates of the prevalence of self-change from addiction to different substances. Recovery from the use of different substances (e.g. tobacco, alcohol, and illicit drugs) and the macro-societal conditions that might promote recovery were also being discussed during this time. Such research, however, was scattered around the globe, and the need for a systematic review of what had been achieved and the identification of future research priorities became more evident.

In March of 1999 the first international conference on *'Natural history of addiction: Recovery from alcohol/tobacco and other drug problems without treatment'* was held at Les Diablerets, Switzerland. The conference, which occurred under the umbrella of the *Kettil Bruun Society for Social and Epidemiological Research on Alcohol (KBS)*, was sponsored by the *Swiss Federal Office of Public Health*, and

1

hosted and organized by the *Swiss Institute for the Prevention of Alcohol and Other Drug Problems*. The conference brought together 29 researchers from more than 10 countries who shared a common interest in self-change/natural recovery. Sociologists, psychologists, health care practitioners, anthropologists, economists, epidemiologists and government policy analysts formed a truly interdisciplinary research group. At the conference the following themes were discussed: (a) natural recovery rates in cross-national comparisons and cultural aspects of change; (b) life event research limits and new directions; (c) implications of research findings for therapeutic interventions; (d) gender and minority factors in natural recovery; (e) a critical assessment of theories of change; (f) group-situation-society, contextual conditions of change; and (g) the use of computer assisted content analysis to bring qualitative and quantitative approaches together. The 'scientific output' of this meeting led to a topical issue which is in press with the journal *Substance Use and Misuse* as well as a miniseries which has been published in the journal *Addiction* [2000;95:747–89].

What made this meeting different from many others was the explicit objective to start a dialogue between researchers, treatment providers, and policy-makers and to gain a clearer vision of the treatment implications in this area. During the meeting a workshop involving physicians and a panel discussion on recommendations were also organized. Taken together, the scientific review of the state of the art on the study of self-change from various disciplines and the rich outcome of the panel discussions with researchers, health care providers, and policy-makers provided the initial framework for this book. Thanks to the personal interest and initiative of Dr. Rihs-Middel of the Swiss Federal Office of Public Health, the conference participants were challenged 'to connect our empirical findings with the world of practice.'

This volume began by the rich interchange of ideas and discussions at the conference. All conference presenters impacted this book. After the conference many participants and a few other individuals working in this area were asked to draft different chapters. The authors listed in this book are the individuals who provided the working materials that constituted the first draft of this book. The work in this volume is truly a collective effort. In the process of editing the book we realized that lines of thought and results could and should be merged across the original individual chapter lines. The generous permission of our colleagues enabled us to work with the manuscript as a whole and mold it into the current volume.

This book on the process of self-change from substance abuse is the first of its kind and is unique as it presents more than research findings. Rather, it presents the process of self-change from several different perspectives – environmental, cross-cultural, preventive – and interventions at both an individual and a societal level. It provides strategies and suggestions for how health care practitioners and government policy-makers alike can aid and foster self-change.

The book is divided into 10 chapters, an introduction/foreword, and an appendix. Chapter 1 begins with an historical overview of the phenomenon of self-change. It reviews conceptual and methodological issues, presents a state-of-the-art review of the field of self-change, and discusses barriers to treatment as well as the major models of change. Chapter 2 provides a comprehensive review of the oft-cited classic alcohol and drug studies of self-change, many of which were not designed to study self-change explicitly, but nevertheless have provided the early base documenting the existence of the phenomenon. Chapter 3 looks at what we know about self-change from substance abuse from large-scale population surveys and community studies as well as from smaller samples obtained by advertising and other means. The advantages and disadvantages of using various methods are discussed as well as questions that are still unanswered about self-change in large populations. Chapter 4 reviews what is known about the self-change process for recovered cigarette smokers and gamblers. Chapter 5 examines the self-change process from a very different perspective. Too often, decisional processes of self-change are seen as occurring within the individual or from interactions between individuals rather than from societal forces. This chapter sets out to show links between the individual clinical view and social factors (e.g. public images of addiction, treatment systems, the role of the media and policy measures) as macro-societal aspects that are of interest to policy-makers. Chapter 6 suggests that while the traditional model would have us believe that there is only one way to resolve addictive behavior, there are '50 ways to leave your lover' or, put differently, multiple pathways to change. The chapter talks about the role of treatment in changing addictive behavior and concludes with the suggestion that one way of providing services efficiently would be for health care practitioners in the substance abuse field to embrace a stepped care model of service provision.

Chapter 7 is a very utilitarian chapter. In the light of what is known about the self-change process, it asks the inevitable question of where health care practitioners fit in. Based on the state of the art, this chapter offers real and practical suggestions about how health-care practitioners can expedite or nurture what might be seen as a time-delayed 'natural' process. By the use of an analogy, a suggestion is made that health care practitioners might take a lesson from farmers, who enhance the natural planting processes and their resultant yield by planting at the right time and by knowing when to apply water and fertilizers. Chapter 8, in discussing the fact that the majority of substance abusers will never cross the clinical threshold (i.e. never enter treatment), offers alternative, nontraditional ways to motivate substance abusers to change (e.g. Internet; self-change material available other than through nontraditional avenues). Chapter 9 expands the discussion of self-change from addiction through an examination of the broader environmental factors that play an important role in substance abusers' recovery. It looks at the powerful effects of environmental influences on the self-change process and in doing so argues that environmental factors are amenable to manipulation to reduce problem use and to promote recovery. Chapter 10 presents information about alcohol and drug use from a broad range of cultural settings and raises important issues and questions. This unique and rich discussion of self-change across different cultures raises many more questions than it answers and reminds us of the importance of differences between cultures.

We also felt that our interview partners should not be treated merely as research subjects or respondents. They, too, should have a say in this book. Therefore, using original interview transcripts, we had the unique opportunity to mirror our scientific statements with the words, sentiments, and feelings of our respondents about how they recovered on their own. Throughout the book boxed excerpts from our respondents are juxtaposed and matched to various discussions about the self-change process. Lastly, we have included an Appendix or 'Toolbox', which is intended as a reference source with 'tips and tools' and other information for researchers, health care practitioners, government analysts, and anyone else interested in the self-change process.

Our hope is that this book with its 'toolbox' will be used as a reference manual by researchers, health care practitioners, public health specialists, and alcohol and drug policy-makers to further understand and promote the self-change process. Although the last decade has witnessed an increased interest in, and understanding of, the study of self-change, our understanding is by no means complete. Thus, the often-heard phrase that 'more research is needed' is relevant to the area of self-change with substance abusers and problem gamblers.

Finally, it is hoped that this book will better inform funding agencies and scientists about where the research 'dollar' or 'euro' is likely to get its best value. In summary, with the publication of this book we are standing on the shoulders of many others.

Harald K. Klingemann and
Linda C. Sobell
Lausanne and Fort Lauderdale
May 2000

REFERENCES

1. Institute of Medicine. (1990) *Broadening the Base of Treatment for Alcohol Problems*, National Academy Press: Washington, DC.
2. American Psychiatric Association. (1994) *Diagnostic and Statistical Manual of Mental Disorders*, 4th ed. American Psychiatric Association: Washington, D.C.

Chapter one

The phenomenon of self-change: overview and conceptual issues

We should also consider those who have a more fleeting contact with deviance, whose careers lead them away from it into conventional ways of life. Thus, for example, studies of delinquents who fail to become adult criminals might teach us even more than studies of delinquents who progress in crime [1, pp. 24–25].

INTRODUCTION

Forty years ago in his classic treatise on the study of deviants Becker [1] cautioned against studying only extreme cases. Over the years other researchers have made similar arguments with regard to studying the addictions. For example, Cahalan [2], based on epidemiological surveys of problem drinkers [3–5], used the term 'tip of the iceberg' to refer to the fact that the survey data demonstrated that clinically defined 'alcoholics' constitute only a relatively small proportion of those whose drinking creates significant problems for themselves and society. Room [6] later labeled this distinction between alcohol problems seen in surveys versus clinical studies as the 'two worlds of alcoholism'. A few years later, based on his well-known longitudinal study, Vaillant [7] asserted that we cannot understand the natural history of alcoholism by looking only at clinic samples. And a decade later, based on a study of Vietnam veterans who used heroin in Vietnam but stopped using it when they returned to the United States, Robins stated that 'Addiction looks very different if you study it in a general population than if you study it in treated cases' [8, p. 1051]. With regard to cocaine, Erickson [9] studied naturally recovered cocaine abusers and concluded that cocaine addicts in treatment represented the tip of the iceberg of all cocaine users. Finally, several other major surveys [10–16] add support to

Cahalan and his colleagues' original findings that treated alcohol and drug abusers constitute only a small percentage of all individuals with such problems.

For years, the addiction field has been dominated by an almost exclusive focus on individuals who are severely dependent. The emphasis on severe dependence has resulted in a myopic view of substance abuse problems that has characterized them as progressive, irreversible, and only resolved through treatment. Further support that the traditional view is myopic comes from studies that shothat those who recover on their own typically have a less serious substance use problem and more intact social resources (e.g. marriages, education, jobs) than those who have sought formal treatment/help [7, 17–21].

If substance use problems are viewed as lying along a continuum ranging from no problems to mild problems to severe problems, rather than as dichotomous (i.e. alcoholic vs. not alcoholic; drug addict vs. not drug addict), this has profound implications for how we view and treat such individuals. One implication is that there are multiple pathways to recovery, including self-change, a pathway that has largely been ignored by the addiction field.

Although there are 10 chapters in this book, this first chapter has several objectives, most notably to help readers understand where the field is and where it is headed. It provides an historical overview of the phenomenon of self-change, it reviews conceptual and methodological issues, it presents a state-of-the-art review of the field of self-change, and it discusses barriers to treatment as well as the major models of change.

THE RESPONDENTS SPEAK

Several investigators who have examined the self-change process with sub-stance abusers have reported that such individuals 'wanted to tell' their stories [21–23]. In this regard, we decided to use respondents' stories to illustrate aspects of the self-change process throughout this book. Thus, starting with this chapter quotations from individuals who were interviewed about their success-ful self-change from addictive behavior are presented in boxes throughout the book. These short narratives relate to various topics discussed within each chapter. The narratives are not meant to be in-depth descriptions of the entire recovery episode and details of the respondents are not provided. Rather, they are included to give readers a grassroots flavor of various issues relating to recovery (e.g. reasons for change; barriers to treatment; maintenance factors) discussed in each chapter. The narratives come from studies of self-change conducted by several of the authors of this book (i.e. D. Finfgeld, W. Cloud, R. Granfield, D. Hodgins, H. Klingemann, L. Sobell, M. Sobell and J. Tucker).

'Telling My Story'

In one of the first studies to comment on respondents' reactions to discussing their self-change from alcohol problems Tuchfeld [23] found alcohol abusers to be quite proud of their recovery without formal help or treatment. Some years later Shaffer and Jones [22] after interviewing cocaine abusers who quit on their own reported that the 'typical cocaine quitter wanted – even felt compelled – to tell us his or her story' (p. 6). Sobell and her colleagues [21] further reported that many recovered alcohol abusers said they had never talked with others about their recovery. Thus, it appears self-changers from substance use problems find the interview experience helpful or therapeutic.

IS WHAT WE CALL THE PHENOMENON IMPORTANT?

Such concepts as 'spontaneous remission', 'natural recovery' and 'maturing out' are not new. In the medical field the term 'spontaneous' has been used for many years and means an improvement in the patient's condition that occurs without treatment [24]. Psychological working definitions [25, 26] of the terms emphasise the individual's own cognitive achievement (i.e. self-initiated recovery or change in behavior). From a sociological viewpoint, the primary consideration is to exit from a deviant career without formal intervention [27] or to mobilise external resources (i.e. self-organised remission) [28]. Lastly, from the perspective of juvenile delinquency the term 'maturing out' has been synonymous with no longer engaging in delinquent behavior [29].

In the addiction field, over the years, several terms (e.g. spontaneous remission, auto-remission, self-change, natural resolution, maturing out, burning out, spontaneous recovery, natural recovery, untreated remission, untreated recovery, auto-remission, self-quitters, spontaneous resolution) have been used to describe individuals who have recovered from addiction on their own (i.e. without formal help or treatment). Although these terms have been used interchangeably, presumably to describe the same phenomenon (i.e. self-change), the notion of spontaneous remission has been challenged as semantically and conceptually imprecise [22, 23, 30, 31]. For example, Mulford has suggested that 'spontaneous remission' is a euphemism for our ignorance of the forces at work' [32, p. 330]. Although some terms used to describe natural recovery suggest the change has no cause, it is doubtful that any investigator of the phenomenon would view it as 'unexplainable', just 'unexplained'.

Lastly, while there is no current agreed upon term, what all these terms have in common is that they suppose that an *unwanted* condition is overcome without professional treatment or help. Words such as *natural* and *spontaneous* increasingly are being replaced by more neutral terms like *untreated recovery* or *self-change*. While the various terms noted above have been used interchangeably to refer to a change in a person's substance use in the absence of formal help or treatment, the preferred term that will be used throughout this book will be *'self-change'*.

DEFINING TREATMENT

Although determining whether treatment has taken place would seem to be a straightforward matter, how treatment episodes are defined in the literature is very fluid. Further, with respect to treatment intensity (i.e. number of sessions), there are other problems. For example, do brief interventions, often involving a single session and sometimes lasting less than 30 minutes, constitute formal treatment [33–36]? Further complicating the picture is advice by lay persons such as ministers, rabbis, and friends. In addition, do we consider community interventions that address change at a broad, social level as treatment (e.g. community- or organization-based smoking-cessation or weight-loss programs that track cumulative results for the community)? A perfect example is the Community Intervention Trial (COMMIT) for Smoking Cessation, a multicenter comprehensive smoking intervention [37–39]. COMMIT was designed to reach cigarette smokers, and to help them achieve and maintain long-term cessation of cigarette smoking through communities, using existing media channels, public education activities, work site activities, major organizations, and social institutions capable of influencing smoking behavior in large groups of people [39, 40].

Mixing treated and untreated respondents

A serious methodological problem with self-change studies in the addiction field has been the mixing of individuals who had received prior treatment with those who never had treatment [20, 21]. Examples of such studies are abundant in the literature [23, 27, 31, 41, 42]. Most of these studies are older and did not subscribe to a strict definition of 'no treatment' and therefore individuals who were unsuccessfully treated but later resolved a drinking problem on their own were included in the study sample. For example, 22% of Tuchfeld's [23, 31] respondents had at some time received treatment for their alcohol problem. To address this problem, some recent self-change studies have presented data separately for individuals who had gone to treatment or self-help meetings several years prior to their recovery but said they recovered on their own, and for self-changers who had no prior treatment or self-help contact [43, 44]. Lastly, it is important to differentiate recovered respondents who have and have not received treatment, for several studies have shown that untreated recovered alcohol abusers and smokers differ from alcohol abusers and smokers who seek treatment in that the untreated groups show less severe problem histories [19, 21, 45–48]. Several studies have also found that untreated recovered alcohol and drug abusers showed greater pre-resolution social stability or had greater social resources than abusers who received treatment.

How little treatment is treatment?

Recent self-change studies [44, 49–55] have addressed the problem of how little treatment is treatment by adopting a conservative definition of treatment, i.e. any intervention by recognized programs or individuals whose primary goal was to treat individuals with substance use problems (e.g. outpatient/inpatient facilities; anti-substance-use drugs; self-help groups attended by respondents to address their own problems; professional counseling specifically for substance use problems; treatment-oriented drinking-driver courses). Because brief interventions for substance abusers have been found to be effective, even one session can be considered treatment. In a related regard, recognizing that a great many individuals might attend a few self-help group meetings without seriously adopting a recovery program, some natural-recovery studies have included respondents who had attended one or two self-help group meetings [21, 44, 56].

An interesting dilemma occurs when one considers the perspective of treatment from different cultures. For example, one recent self-change study defined the absence of treatment as no more than five outpatient visits with a physician [57]. The reason is that in Germany, where the research was conducted, alcohol treatment until very recently took the form of psychiatric hospitalization and five outpatient visits (which is more than enough to qualify as a brief intervention) and this seemed to the investigators not to constitute treatment.

Another issue that has clouded this area of research is that many have confused research like Vaillant's, which describes the *natural history of change* across the life span (i.e. looking at the progression of the disorder or help-seeking, including treatment and self-help group use), with *natural recovery in the absence of treatment or self-help groups* [58, 59].

STATE OF THE ART IN SELF-CHANGE

Although self-change outcomes in the areas of substance abuse have been identified since the 1960s [60–62], research on self-change has recently experienced a resurgence [12, 19, 44]. Surprisingly, though, the study of self-change has been very uneven across the addiction field. While it is a documented and common route to recovery for cigarette smokers (estimates range from 80% to 90% of all those who stop smoking; [63–68], until the past decade the systematic study of self-change has been largely ignored for alcohol and other drugs [20]. In this regard, a recent review of the literature found only 38 alcohol and drug studies published or in press through 1997 that met methodological inclusion criteria [20]. For other addictive behaviors such as specific eating disorders [61, 69–71] and gambling [17, 72] there is a dearth of studies examining self-change.

Finally, while this book focuses on studies of natural recovery from addictive behavior, such recovery has also been reported for other clinical problems. For example, self-change has been the subject of previous studies of neuroses [73] and stuttering [74, 75]. In fact, the majority of 'psychological' problems people experience are not brought to the attention of mental health professionals or paraprofessionals [76]. Instead, problems generally are shared with 'natural helpers' who possess no mental health training [77].

While methodologically rigorous studies of natural recovery from addictive behavior are relatively new [20], published studies and isolated reports are not new. One of the earliest reports was in the early 19th century by Benjamin Rush [78], a distinguished physician and author of one of the earliest scientific treatises on inebriety. He described several individuals who had recovered from alcohol problems on their own (alcohol treatment as we know it today was non-existent in the 1800s). Further, some of these individuals even appeared to have become moderate drinkers (i.e. they gave up the evils of 'spirituous liquors').

Since 1975 several reviews of self-change from substance abuse have been published [66, 79–86]. The early literature, however, added little to our under-standing of natural recovery other than to suggest that there is considerable variability in the types of life-event associated with natural recovery [20]. In addition, most of the identified life-events were global in nature (e.g. changes in family milieu, friends, vocation, health, religion, or social pressure). Part of the reason that we know so little is that the design of most of the early studies was exploratory in nature [82] and methodologically flawed [20, 21].

Evidence for self-change from addictive behavior comes from several lines of study:

(a)   prevalence and longitudinal (i.e. cases identified at two different points in time) studies in the general population [3, 4, 19, 87];

(b)   waiting-list control groups [88, 89] or follow-up of clients who left treatment [90];

(c)   active case-finding methods include studies that specifically recruited and interviewed individuals who have recovered without formal help or treatment [17, 22, 25, 31, 41, 44, 56]; case finding largely has been done through media advertisements [44, 49, 55] and snowballing (i.e. nomination of someone that the respondent knows has a problem similar to the his/her's) [91, 92] techniques [20]; and

(d)   official registers of addicts [62, 93].

Advantages of survey and other methods for studying self-change

Although surveys have many advantages over other methods for studying self-change, there are some disadvantages as well. Surveys usually involve large samples of the general population and hence can provide overall rates of self-change. However, most surveys contain very few, if any, questions about the actual process of self-change. On the other hand, studies using snowballing techniques or selected advertising to recruit recovered substance abusers typically focus on recovery issues and how recovery proceeds.

WHY HAS SELF-CHANGE AS AN AREA OF STUDY BEEN SO LONG OVERLOOKED OR IGNORED?

For many years the addiction field either paid little attention to or ignored self-change as an area of study [21, 22], and it was even considered a taboo topic by some [94]. The idea that someone with an addiction can overcome the problem without extensive professional help was, and to some extent still is, met with disbelief by many health care professionals as well as the general public [95–99]. Another reason why self-change has been ignored as an area of inquiry may relate to the fact that individuals who exhibit severe forms of the disorder have occupied public attention. Lastly, researchers and clinicians seldom encounter people who recover on their own. Thus, many in the field are blind to the fact that there are multiple pathways to recovery (e.g. treatment, self-help groups like AA, self-change).

A third and salient reason why natural recovery has long been ignored relates to the disease model of addiction [20, 22, 94, 98]. The disease model not only has long dominated the field, but also is an approach that is wholly inconsistent with self-change. Advocates of the disease model put forth a tautological argument that 'an ability to cease addictive behaviors on one's own suggests that the individual was not addicted in the first place. If one is *not* able to stop independently, then an addiction is present' [94, p. 306]. As reflected in the three quotes in the next box, the disease model proponents postulate a progressive irreversible disorder that can only be resolved through intervention.

Attitudes similar to those noted above are also found in the sociological labelling approach, which for a long time focused on the progressive consolidation of deviant careers and viewed the individual as a victim of stigmatisation by the agencies of social control [102, 103]. Not only has such thinking led to an assumption that people with substance use disorders cannot recover on their own, but some have suggested that failure to seek treatment for a substance abuse problem will have fatal consequences.

Another issue that runs counter to the disease model of addiction is the claim that individuals can engage in low-risk drinking or drug use (also referred to as chipping, see [22]). Studies showing that this is possible have over the years

---

Traditionalists Claim Self-Change is Not Possible

'Addiction is not selfcuring. Left alone addiction only gets worse, leading to total degradation, to prison, and, ultimately to death' [100, p. xixii].

'Alcoholism is a fatal disease, 100 percent fatal. Nobody survives alcoholism that remains unchecked ... these people will not be able to stop drinking by themselves. They are forced to seek help; and when they don't, they perish miserably' [101, p. 1].

'There has been considerable skepticism in both lay and professional circles of the thesis that many addicts never stop using drugs, but continue as addicts until they die ...' [62, p.1].

---

been met with emotional reactions ranging from deep-seated lack of belief to serious attacks [104–108]. Thus, studies reporting that naturally recovered alcohol and drug abusers have successfully returned to low-risk non-problem alcohol or drug use are seen as a dual threat to the disease model (i.e. recovering without treatment and reversing the disorder). Interestingly, as will be discussed shortly, a recent review of the self-change literature found low-risk alcohol and drug use to be frequent [20].

In summary, although the concept of self-change runs counter to the disease model of addiction and has been met with disbelief, there has been a significant increase in research in this area in the past decade [20]. Further, self-change from substance abuse has been gaining recognition and acceptance by prestigious bodies such as, in the United States, the Institute of Medicine [30] and the American Psychiatric Association [109].

WHY STUDY THE SELF-CHANGE PROCESS?

Several notable addiction researchers have suggested that much can be gained by studying the self-change process. For example, over a quarter of a century ago, Orford and Edwards [110] insightfully urged that 'the way ahead in alcoholism treatment research should be to embrace more closely the study of 'natural forces' that can then be captured and exploited by planned interventions' (p. 3). Vaillant [111] also suggested that 'if treatment as we currently understand it does not seem more effective than natural healing processes, then we need to understand those healing processes' (p. 18).

One of the several compelling reasons for studying natural recovery is the fact that the substance abuse field does not have enduring effective treatments [112–114]. Not one treatment can be pointed to as having demonstrated a high rate of sustained recovery. Also, little is known about how to successfully match individuals to treatment [115–117]. In addition, an understanding of the self-change process could be used to design more effective treatment programs [44, 85, 87, 110], and alert professionals to the need to consider contextual inflluences on the recovery process [53, 54, 118]. Studies that gathered data on the reasons for natural recovery, although few in number, have begun to shed some light on what might trigger and maintain the recovery process [20].

A third reason for studying the self-change process is, as mentioned earlier, that the vast majority of individuals with alcohol, drug, and smoking problems never come to the attention of researchers or clinicians, as they never seek treatment. For example, in the alcohol field the ratio of untreated to treated alcohol abusers has been estimated to range from 3:1 to 13:1 [24, 119], and over three-quarters of ex-smokers are self-quitters [64, 65, 120]. For gambling, it is estimated that less than 3% of all those diagnosed as pathological gamblers (i.e. most severe cases) have received treatment [121].

Stigma and Embarrassment: A Big Barrier

Respondent A: 'Yes, because I think people usually look at alcoholics as down and outers, you know. And a person that's just a social drinker doesn't want to be associated with those kinds. Like the ones you see down in the lower end of the city, these winos. That's what you class yourself as a true alcoholic'.

Respondent B: 'I think the strongest one was the embarrassment before my relatives and my friends that I had to go to AA or some other place. If I had gone to go those places I was admitting or letting everybody say that I was an alcoholic and to this day I don't think I was an alcoholic. I think I had a heavy drinking problem'.

Respondent C: 'I don't think anybody want's to be classified as an alcoholic or a drunk rummy. At least I didn't. I was embarrassed, yes'.

Respondent D: 'I don't feel I'm an alcoholic period. I have a ... I had a drinking problem but the word is terrible'.

Respondent E: 'Because I'm a maybe a private person I wasn't the type that, you know, would go out and seek help and I would be embarrassed if a lot of people were ... heard about the problem'.

The literature shows that substance abusers have reported three major reasons for not entering conventional treatment programs (a) the stigma associated with being labeled, (b) substance abusers' beliefs that their problems are not serious enough to warrant attention (i.e. conventional programs are often too intense and too demanding for individuals who are not severely dependent), and (c) substance abusers want to handle their problem on their own [17, 20, 72, 94, 122].

Doing It On My Own: Why I Did Not Seek Formal Help or Treatment

Respondent A: ' I just felt that if I couldn't do it on my own a group of people isn't going to help me at all. A very good friend of mine he just got his ten year pin so ... He's very proud of it and he should be but I just couldn't ... They are friends of mine but I just couldn't. If I can't quit by myself I just didn't see how anyone else was going to help me. I have nothing against AA don't misunderstand me, it's a good organization but 15 to 20 people aren't' going to tell me what to do'.

Respondent B: 'I felt I had a problem but I didn't figure I was like over the edge sort of thing and I figured it wasn't bad enough that I couldn't cure it myself'.

Respondent C: 'Well I think I had the feeling that if I'm gonna beat this thing, it's up to me, and nobody else is going to make me stop drinking. It's my problem and I have to resolve it myself. Why should I go to, and ask somebody else and put my problems on their shoulders, when it's one of my own'.

Respondent D: 'I guess self pride like I didn't feel ... I wanted to try it without it. I think I may have gone to AA perhaps or some agency if I hadn't have been able to beat it myself but initially I just wanted to do it on my own and thought I could'.

Respondent E: 'Only that I think it's a greater victory because I did it on my own. I didn't need anybody else'.

Other barriers have included non-availability of treatment, negative attitudes toward treatment, or that treatment was too costly [17, 20, 21, 49, 122]. The critical point with respect to stigmatization and other barriers to treatment is that they cannot be completely understood by studying only treated individuals.

More Barriers to Treatment

Money

Respondent A: 'This decision about you know it took a lot of money you don't ... about going to get outside help, now that would have been beyond my personal with my salary scale. Now that was out pretty well'.

Respondent B: 'Well yes because I couldn't afford some of this jazz about going to a sanatorium and I could not afford that'.

Attitude Toward Treatment

Respondent A: 'Well, I wasn't all that sold on the idea that any of these treatment centers could help you'.

Respondent B: 'I have a poor opinion of the medical profession. I have a poor opinion of all the experts not just medical'.

Lack of Facilities

Respondent A: 'I'm not aware of them (i.e. treatment facilities). The only one I can think of is probably AA'.

Respondent B: 'I guess really not being aware of any treatment facilities'.

BARRIERS TO TREATMENT/HELP SEEKING FOR RACIAL/ETHNIC MINORITIES AND WOMEN

Studies that have looked at barriers to entering alcohol treatment [44, 46, 51, 123–128] have generally found that a variety of specific barriers confront individuals who seek treatment or who have never entered treatment (e.g. stigma associated with an alcohol problem, not recognizing a problem, cultural differences, geography, financial issues, need for child care). Several studies have also found significant gender differences in reports of barriers to treatment [129-134].

One study [135] that examined differences among problem drinkers in treatment and in the general population found important differences in the factors that influence treatment entry for women (e.g. lifetime general treatment history, ethnicity, employment) and men (e.g. social consequences, treatment history, employment). In another study looking at gender differences, Weisner [136] found that female were more likely than male problem drinkers to use non-alcohol-specific health care settings, particularly mental health treatment services, and to report greater symptom severity. Others have similarly found that women seek non-traditional avenues of help such as general health and mental health care settings for dealing with their alcohol problems [132, 137, 138].

It is likely that the availability and acceptance of professional help and treatment also influence the rates of natural recovery. According to Duckert [139], the failure of treatment systems to adapt to the specific needs of female addicts and 'the lack of more attractive treatment alternatives' (p. 176) are major reasons for the apparent relative unwillingness of women to seek treatment. Therefore, natural recovery would be expected to occur more frequently among women than among men, because women can do less about their problem.

Alcohol Abuse a Worse Stigma for Women

Respondent A: 'I feel that to be labeled an alcoholic, especially as a woman, is degrading and it means you're something kind of like . . . you don't have any willpower. You make an ass of yourself. It's sort of disgusting to me'

Respondent B: 'Yes too embarrassing. Especially . . . it's always ok for a man to drink and it's great for a man to seek help but as a woman, you look . . . it's not quite the same thing'.

Respondent C: 'I didn't want to be found out. I didn't . . . because I still think, perhaps it's not quite so much now but it is more of a stigma for a woman'.

Given the lower prevalence of problem drinking among women than among men [140] and that among heroin addicts there is a typical male-female ratio of 4:1 [141], small absolute numbers of female respondents are to be expected in self-change studies. Treatment specialists frequently attribute the relatively low number of women substance abusers in treatment not to the inadequacy of treatment for women's' needs but to the stigma attached to female drunkenness or heroin addiction [142]. As regards illicit-drug users, an additional gender-specific bias may result from using snowball sampling techniques, as such procedures favor gender-specific communication networks in the drug scene, and thus, they favor the inclusion of males.

In a recent review of naturally recovered alcohol and drug abusers, the mean percentage of women across all studies was 31.6% [20], a figure only slightly higher than figures for alcohol treatment facilities where a quarter of the clients are female [143]. The fact that about one-third of all alcohol and drug abusers who naturally recover are female is consistent with results from brief courses of treatment to which larger than expected samples of females are recruited through advertisements [48, 144].

A few studies have looked at gender differences in studies of self-change [51, 53, 128, 145], and have generally found an absence of significant variables as a function of gender in both treated and untreated samples of opiate and alcohol abusers. One plausible reason is that both brief treatments and self-change embody the concept of greater empowerment and thus are more appealing to women than entering traditional addiction treatment programs which are not only viewed as more stigmatizing but also promote a disease-based sense of powerlessness.

In contrast to the sizeable body of literature in the addiction field examining and identifying factors that affect treatment entry by gender there are 'very few studies that inform differences in service use by ethnicity' [138, p. 79]. Though access to treatment for minorities has not been widely evaluated, there is evidence that such factors as lack of health insurance and a greater likelihood of living below the poverty level limit access to treatment for Hispanics and African-American [146].

In an excellent review of ethnic and cultural minority groups, Castro and his colleagues [147] found that (a) past studies have shown that minority clients have questioned seeking mental health and substance abuse services from mainstream agencies; (b) there is a high dropout rate among minority clients who seek counseling; it has been suggested that one reason for this high dropout rate is that counselors are not culturally empathic [148]; and (c) failure to engage clients in treatment either through rapport or raising positive expectations have been factors suggested as likely to affect dropouts. A further reason for failure to enter treatment and for high dropout is that most substance abuse treatment programs have neither been designed nor evaluated for minorities.

Because of the stigma associated with entering alcohol treatment generally, coupled with the reluctance of women and minorities to enter mainstream substance abuse programs, self-change studies and interventions for these two groups are critical. Furthermore, cross-cultural comparisons of self-change within and between countries are needed to determine generalizability of findings. Lastly, while national surveys have shown treatment utilization to vary by gender and ethnic groups, this may be due to any one of several factors (e.g. agency discrimination, lack of interest, failure to recognize a problem, unattractiveness of available services or non-existent services). Thus, one issue for the development of alternative services is to be sensitive to the needs of particular groups and individuals. The old adage of one size fits all is clearly outdated.

MODELS OF CHANGE

Over the past 35 years several models of change or models of decisional processes have been posited. Although the models span more than three decades, they all have inherent similarities. Although this chapter is not the forum in which to review these models in depth, a brief description of the prevailing models will help set the context for the studies and findings reported in subsequent chapters. At the heart of the decisional theories of behavior change is an inherent cost-benefit evaluation which is cognitively based. These theories look at beliefs and feelings and their role in how decisions to change behavior occur. What drives an addiction is that initially and perhaps for some time the pluses outweigh the minuses [149]. Over time, addicts weigh the positives and negatives of their use and when they perceive that the negatives outweigh the positives they then are more likely to decide to stop or reduce their use.

In a seminal research article, Eysenck [150] questioned the effectiveness of psychotherapy for what was then called neurosis. Reviewing treatment studies published up to that time, Eysenck concluded that 'roughly two-thirds of a group of neurotic patients will recover or improve to a marked extent within about two years of the onset of their illness' (p. 322). By virtue of his early questioning of the effectiveness of psychotherapy Eysenck was also one of the first to try to understand what were the common elements of therapeutic change for behavior and mental health problems. From that time forward, several comprehensive models of change have been proposed that integrate different theoretical models of the change process [151].

Conflict theory

Janis and Mann's [152] conflict theory postulates that tension results when there is dissonance between attitudes. To reduce dissonance, individuals must examine the positive and negative aspects of conflicting viewpoints and make a decision about how to lessen the conflict. Janis and Mann's decision-making model involves five stages of decision-making: (a) appraisal of a challenge, (b) appraisal of alternatives, (c) selection of the best alternative, (d) commitment to the new policy, and (e) adherence to the new policy despite negative feedback [152, 153]. An individual's effort to resolve tension (i.e. inner conflict) is thought to be a function of the amount of dissonance between beliefs.

Transtheoretical model of change

The transtheoretical model of change grew out of efforts to apply a set of common change processes from existing theories of therapy to the process of smoking cessation. In explaining behavior change, Prochaska and DiClemente [154] use a five-stage model of change (i.e. precontemplation, contemplation, preparation, action, and maintenance) similar to the decision-making stages put forth by Janis and Mann [152]. Prochaska and DiClemente's model, however, applies to change outside of therapy [155] and asserts that the stage of change in which people are reflects the likelihood of their changing [156]. In this model, (a) precontemplators are individuals who are not considering changing; (b) contemplators are thought to be considering change; (c) preparation occurs when an individual starts to make plans to change; (d) individuals in the action stage are actively engaging in change; (e) people in the maintenance stage are sustaining their change, and lastly; (f) if a change attempt fails, the person is viewed as relapsing, and the stage process starts over again.

Crystallization of discontent

Baumeister [157] has conceptualized the change process as related to a person's personal perception of circumstances surrounding his/her behavior. He further asserts that people continually re-evaluate their beliefs and behavior in an effort to maintain consistency while maintaining their beliefs. In this process, individuals make attributions that support their choices. Using examples from marriage and religion, Baumeister explains how people make extreme causal attributions in an effort to support the commitments or beliefs they hold. He posits that people also discount disconfirming evidence so as to retain their commitments or beliefs.

Baumeister [157] states that if consequences perceived by the individual as negative reach a threshold of discomfort for the individual, he/she will come to see the consequences as related, thereby crystallizing the belief that the consequences are strongly linked with the behavior. He calls this process 'crystallization of discontent'. Thus, when an individual's perception crystallizes or solidifies negative aspects as related to a belief, affiliation, or behavior, the individual becomes motivated to change the situation. For example, one might end a committed relationship perceived to have become negative as a result of becoming aware of uncomfortable consequences beyond that which the individual is willing to tolerate. Another example would be a change in political beliefs as one comes to realize that the consequences of such beliefs are unacceptable. In the addiction field Winick's [62] maturation hypothesis is a good example of the process of crystallization of discontent. Addicts who quit drugs talk about the extra hustle involved in getting drugs that over time builds such that the negative consequences eventually reach a threshold of discomfort and this feeling of discomfort motivates behavior change (i.e. drug addicts are no longer willing to, or do not have the energy to, continue to do drugs).

Becoming an ex

In a process of change akin to Baumeister's crystallization of discontent, Ebaugh [158] describes the change process as a role exit that includes developing a perception that a current role is not what the individual desired when she/he began the role. She refers to this as 'Becoming an Ex'. A good example of Ebaugh's role exiting involves nuns who after taking their vows and entering the convent start over time to see things they strongly disagree with about church policy. As their disenchantment builds, their commitment in the face of negative consequences (i.e. disagreement with church policy, defrocking) decreases. As the consequences build, dissonance increases between what the individual values and what her role entails. The point where someone finally decides to exit a role and becomes motivated to do something different is seen as a focal point where the person has finally crystallized his/her discontent. Ebaugh [158] feels 'turning points' play an important role in behavior change as they '(a) announce to others and give ultimate reasons for change; (b) reduce cognitive dissonance and conflict; and (c) help mobilize resources (p. 134)'.

Self-change and stages of change (SC) model

In terms of self-change, there is a need to understand where and how these recoveries fit into the self-change model [98]. However, before rushing to explain how self-change recoveries fit into this model, it should be noted that this model has started to come under increasing scrutiny for not adequately accounting for the complexity of behavior change [159–163]. It has been argued that the SC model is a complex way of describing behavior that can better be explained on a continuum, and that change from addictive behavior does not move system-atically through discrete stages [160, 161, 163]. In terms of a true stage-model all stages must be passed through and no stages are revisited [159]. The SC model violates both of these premises because, when people relapse, the model asserts that they must return to an earlier stage. Further, because many who recover on their own do so the first time they decide to stop, this contradicts the model where relapse is a required stage. In this regard, a recent study reported that 42.9% (15/35) of naturally recovered alcohol abusers successfully resolved on their first attempt [164]. Finally, cases of true spontaneous remission (e.g. religion conversions) cannot pass through all stages, jumping instead from precontemplation to action.

Lastly, although the transtheoretical model has received increasing attention over the past decade and has inspired much of the empirical work on 'Readiness to Change' (RTC), the psychometric literature provides inconsistent support for the stages of change [161]. As with others who have criticised the stages-of-change-model, Carey and her colleagues [161] suggest that RTC (i.e. the degree to which an individual is motivated to change a problem behavior) may best be thought of as a 'multidimensional and continuous construct with complex relationships to behavior, cognition, and environmental content' (p. 245).

MAJOR FINDINGS FROM SELF-CHANGE STUDIES

Although the study of natural recovery is new, the majority of the studies have several findings in common. The major and notable findings from self-change studies are briefly discussed below.

Self-change: A major pathway to recovery

Several major surveys have shown that self-change appears to be the dominant pathway to recovery: (a) cigarettes [64, 65, 67, 68]; (b) alcohol [11, 12, 19, 165]; (c) drugs [165]; and (d) gambling [72]. An excellent example is the well-known National Longitudinal Alcohol Epidemiologic Survey (NLAES), which evaluated shifting drinking patterns in both treated and untreated groups and found that the vast majority of alcohol dependent drinkers changed on their own [12].

In terms of self-change studies of alcohol and drug abusers, a recent review [20] found that the majority have been conducted with alcohol abusers (75%; 30/40), with heroin abusers a distant second (22.5%). Lastly, very few self-change studies have been conducted for such drugs as cocaine or marijuana (7.5% and 2.5%, respectively). Finally, the majority of the alcohol and drug abuser self-change studies were conducted in the US, Europe, and Canada (59.1%, 18.9%, and 16.2%, respectively; [20]).

Can we believe what they tell us?

Corroboration of self-changers' self-reports is important because respondents are being asked to recall events over long time-periods. As with treated substance abusers, the primary confirmation of the self-reports of self-changers has been by interviewing collaterals and through official records [reviewed in 20].

Studies which examined the validity of self-reports among naturally recovered substance abusers [21, 44, 56, 79, 166–169] have found that these individuals give reasonably accurate accounts of their pre- and post-recovery substance use when compared with similar reports from their collaterals. The results parallel findings from studies of treated substance abusers [170–174]. Although some studies [44, 49, 164] have reported problems in getting respondents to provide the name of someone who knew them when they had their problem (i.e. in the distant past, e.g. 10–20 years ago), one suggestion has been to incorporate reliability checks (e.g. ask the same questions when first screened into the project and when interviewed at a later date) into the interview process [20]. Generally, it can be concluded that naturally recovered substance abusers' reports of their pre- and post-recovery and related experiences are consistent with reports from other sources [20, 44, 62, 166, 167].

Stability of natural recovery

A recent review of self-change studies found that across all studies the average recovery length was slightly over six years [20]. Because substance use is a highly recurrent disorder [26] and because several recent studies have suggested that stability of recovery with or without treatment does not seem to occur for at least five years [12, 175–177], it is suggested that studies of the self-change process use a minimum recovery period of five or more years. Such a recovery period parallels findings from the medical field that show that a survival rate of five or more years is associated with very stable outcomes from serious diseases [178, 179].

Longitudinal studies of self-changers can also be used to examine how changes in the use of one substance relates to changes in other behavior. There have been a few reports of respondents stopping one drug but increasing the use of another [25, 174], and one longitudinal study found that close to one-half of naturally recovered alcohol abusers within the first six months of stopping drinking alcohol reported increases in the use of nonalcoholic beverages; a quarter also reported that they ate more sweet things, and about one fifth reported smoking more cigarettes as well as eating more food [177]. However, some studies have found the contrasting finding that cessation of alcohol problems was associated with an increase in likelihood of subsequent smoking cessation [180].

A final issue concerns evaluating the use and abuse of all drugs, not just the substance from which the person recovered. For example, heavy drinking has been reported with some naturally recovered cocaine abusers [49]. In another study, for some naturally recovered heroin addicts who were totally abstinent 'the use of other drugs, especially alcohol, continued for longer periods and eventually became a problem in themselves' [25, p. 126].

Low-risk drinking and drug use outcomes

As discussed above, a central tenet of traditional concepts of alcohol and drug problems is that recovery can only occur through abstinence. Interestingly, a recent review of the self-change literature makes very clear that this aspect of conventional wisdom is inaccurate [20]. In that review, more than three-quarters (78.6%) of the studies of individuals who recovered from alcohol problems reported some low-risk drinking outcomes. As shown in Table 1, two-fifths (40.3%) of all alcohol recoveries involved low-risk drinking, suggesting that low-risk drinking is a common route to recovery among naturally recovered alcohol abusers. These findings parallel those from alcohol treatment outcome studies [181–183] and suggest that the way the field views recovery from alcohol problems is not consistent with the empirical evidence. Lastly, most self-changers with an alcohol problem who return to moderate drinking also appear to have been less dependent on alcohol, a finding similar to that for individuals in alcohol treatment studies who moderate their drinking [108].

Table 1 Route of recovery from alcohol and drugs

Variable	Mean (SD) or mean % across respondent samples	Median	Range
Type of alcohol recovery (*n* = 26)			
Abstinence	59.7%	62.0%	3.0–100%
Low-risk drinking	40.3%	38.0%	0.0–97.0%
Type of drug recovery (*n* = 10)			
Abstinence	85.5%	100.0%	0.0–100%
Limited drug use	14.5%	0%	0.0–100%

Adapted from [20]

Although fewer studies of natural recovery from drug problems as opposed to alcohol problems have been reported, similar post-recovery drug use patterns have emerged with drug abusers. Nearly half (46.2%; *n* = 6) of the drug studies reviewed reported recovery involving limited drug use, and across all drug recoveries, as shown above, 14.5% involved reduced use [20]. In light of the fact that both controlled opiate use [43, 184–188] and cocaine use [189–192] have been reported previously, these results are not surprising.

WHAT TRIGGERS SELF-CHANGE? THINKING ABOUT CHANGING

One of the most common ways that self-change (drugs [25, 41, 44, 49, 50], smoking [63, 91], alcohol [167, 192]) has been reported to occur is by a process described as a 'cognitive appraisal' or a 'cognitive evaluation' (i.e. individuals report that their initiation of change was preceded by a process of their weighing the pros and cons of changing their substance use and eventually becoming committed to change). With the exception of gambling [17], cognitive appraisals have been reported across a variety of substances: (a) cigarettes [63]; (b) drugs such as cocaine and heroin [25, 49, 192, 193]; and (c) alcohol [41, 44, 50, 91, 193]. Further support for a cognitive appraisal process comes from a recent review of the literature [20] where 27.5% of the studies reported such reasons for recovery, while 62.5% reported health-related reasons. Similar cognitive processes have also been reported for treated alcohol abusers with long-term recovery [194]. Collectively, the results from these studies suggest that ongoing cognitive evaluations are *central* to the change process for many individuals who have had problems with alcohol, drugs and cigarettes, but recover on their own.

Recoveries Described as Cognitive Appraisals

Respondent A: 'You know, I had thought about it for a while and I had made up my mind that I wanted to do it. To me, I had a problem. It was a big problem. It was a bigger problem than I certainly thought that I had. And once I came to grips with it and realized that there was something wrong there ... that once I started thinking along those lines, it wasn't too long before I discovered what the problem was and why it was there. So if it's staring you in the face, I mean you got to do something about it ... So I just made up my mind to stop drinking. But this ... didn't happen Tuesday, Thursday or Wednesday ... There's a lot more to it than that. I mean it's hard for me to sit here and tell you how I was thinking Tuesday, 1978. Or how I was thinking Wednesday, but the overall picture ... that's about as plain as I can make it ... how it came about. It was a process of ... over a period of time. It was a gradual thing. It was probably over a year, maybe 18 months time'.

Respondent B: 'I looked at myself as being dirt, that I had not achieved more than that; when you are 36 years old, you begin to draw kind of a balance sheet, you realize you are down on the ground and you have spent everything on alcohol'.

Recovery associated with cognitive evaluations as opposed to recovery precipitated by discrete events is of particular interest as such recovery has implications for clients in treatment as well as for individuals who want to change on their own but do not want to enter treatment [195]. If a cognitive appraisal process (e.g. a balance sheet evaluating the pros and cons of continuing to use and not use) facilitates the resolution of substance abuse problems, then outcomes for clients might be improved by having them engage in an appraisal of their substance use. A decisional balance process has been used successfully with smokers and for weight loss [196, 197] and is currently being evaluated in a large community intervention [195]. However, as several studies have also shown, thinking about changing does not take place in isolation, but is often triggered and influenced by environmental factors, such as changes in the ovreall life context or pressure and/or support from relatives and friends [51–56, 91, 118]. In many cases, positive incentives, exerting their influence against a background of cumulating negative consequences, play an important role in the decisional process [43, 51–53].

MAINTAINING RECOVERY

In terms of coping strategies for maintaining recovery, the literature is scant, but consistent. The biggest factor associated with maintaining recovery has been social support or a positive milieu, particularly from friends and family [20, 23, 43, 44, 63]. These findings are consistent with the literature showing that a positive family milieu or social support is the most notable factor associated with positive outcomes in treatment studies [198, 199].

Resolved Alcohol Abuser

'[I stayed] away from old playmates and the old playground with people who drink and use ... [and stayed] connected with positive people in positive environments'.

For drug abusers, another common strategy for avoiding relapse is to leave the environment where drugs are used and to break off social relationships with friends who use drugs [20, 192].

FUTURE DIRECTIONS

As noted in a recent review of the literature [20], future studies of self-change need to be methodologically sound, and they also need to uniformly report demographic and substance-use-history information. Otherwise, it will be impossible to draw conclusions across substances. In addition, a minimum recovery interval of five or more years has been suggested in order to draw conclusions that are not biased as a result of being based on transient or unstable recovery. It will also be important to identify substance-related differences (e.g. environmental change such as moving may be an important factor in natural recovery from heroin, but less important for alcohol) and commonalities (e.g. social support may be a helpful maintenance factor for all substance abusers). Finally, since one of the goals of studying natural recovery is to understand what factors might be associated with successful recovery and to test those factors in clinical interventions, an in-depth qualitative understanding of what drives and maintains recovery in the absence of treatment or self-help is critical. So far, only a few studies [51, 53, 55, 200] have explicitly compared successful recovery with and without treatment.

In summary, the proliferation of self-change studies in the addiction field and the findings of low-risk alcohol and drug use provide empirical support for a conceptualization of alcohol and drug problems that does not declare progressivity to be a required element of substance-use disorders and that recognizes that there are multiple pathways to recovery, including moderation and harm reduction. As well, the evidence clearly supports that substance abuse problems should be viewed as lying along a continuum from no problems to mild problems to severe problems rather than as a dichotomy. Such a view, of course, has implications for the types and intensities of services than are offered. Lastly, with one exception [201], there have been no investigations of the self-change processes across different cultural or social contexts [98]. Thus, to substantiate that self-change and what triggers it is not culture-specific, cross-cultural evaluations are needed.

REFERENCES

1.   Becker, H.S. (1963) *Outsiders*, Free Press: New York.
2.   Cahalan, D. (1987) *Studying Drinking Problems Rather Than Alcoholism*, Plenum: New York.
3.   Cahalan, D. (1970) *Problem Drinkers: A National Survey*, Jossey-Bass: San Francisco.
4.   Cahalan, D., Cisin, I.H. and Crossley, H.M. *American Drinking Practices*, Rutgers Center of Alcohol Studies: New Brunswick, NJ.
5.   Cahalan, D. and Room, R. (1974) *Problem Drinking Among American Men*, Rutgers Center of Alcohol Studies: New Brunswick, NJ.
6.   Room, R. (1977) *Measurement and Distribution of Drinking Patterns and Problems in General Populations*, Geneva: World Health Organization: Geneva.
7.   Vaillant, G.E. and Milofsky, E.S. (1984) Natural history of male alcoholism: Paths to recovery, in *Longitudinal Research in Alcoholism* (eds D.W. Goodwin, K.T.V. Dusen and S.A. Mednick) Kluwer-Nijhoff Publishing, pp. 53–71.
8.   Robins, L.N. (1993) Vietnam veterans' rapid recovery from heroin addiction: A fluke or normal expectation? *Addiction* 88, 1041–1054.
9.   Erickson, P.G. and Alexander, B.K. (1989) Cocaine and addictive liability. *Soc Pharmacol.* 3, 249–270.
10. Cunningham, J.A. (1999) Untreated remissions from drug use: The predominant pathway. *Addict Behav.* 24(2), 267–270.
11. Cunningham, J.A., Lin, E., Ross, E. and Walsh, G.W. (2000) Factors associated with untreated remissions from alcohol abuse or dependence. *Addict Behav.* 25, 317–321.
12. Dawson, D.A. (1996) Correlates of past-year status among treated and untreated persons with former alcohol dependence: United States, 1992. *Alcohol: Clin Exp Res.* 20, 771–779.
13. Grant, B.F. (1997) Barriers to alcoholism treatment: Reasons for not seeking treatment in a general population sample. *J Stud Alcohol* 58(4), 365–371.
14. Narrow, W.E., Regier, D.A., Rae, D.S., Manderscheid, R.W. and Locke, B.Z. (1993) Use of services by persons with mental and addictive disorders: Findings from the National Institute of Mental Health epidemiologic catchment area program. *Arch Gen Psychiatry* 50, 95–107.
15. Roizen, R. (1977) *Barriers to Alcoholism Treatment*, Alcohol Research Group: Berkeley, CA.

16. Room, R. and Greenfield, T. (1993) Alcoholics Anonymous, other 12 step movements and psychotherapy in the United States population, 1990. *Addiction* **88**, 555–562.
17. Hodgins, D.C. and El-Guebaly, N. (2000) Natural and treatment-assisted recovery from gambling problems: A comparison of resolved and active gamblers. *Addiction* **95**, 777–789.
18. Humphreys, K., Moos, R.H. and Finney, J.W. Two pathways out of drinking problems without professional treatment. *Addict Behav.* **20**(4), 427–441.
19. Sobell, L.C., Cunningham, J.A. and Sobell, M.B. (1996) Recovery from alcohol problems with and without treatment: Prevalence in two population surveys. *Am J Public Health* **86**(7), 966–972.
20. Sobell, L.C., Ellingstad, T.P. and Sobell, M.B. (2000) Natural recovery from alcohol and drug problems: Methodological review of the research with suggestions for future directions. *Addiction* **95**, 749–769.
21. Sobell, L.C., Sobell, M.B. and Toneatto, T. (1992) Recovery from alcohol problems without treatment, in *Self-control and the Addictive Behaviours* (eds. N. Heather, W.R. Miller and J. Greeley), Maxwell MacMillan: New York.
22. Shaffer, H.J. and Jones, S.B. (1989) *Quitting Cocaine: The Struggle Against Impulse*, Lexington Books: Lexington, MA.
23. Tuchfeld, B.S. (1981) Spontaneous remission in alcoholics: Empirical observations and theoretical implications. *J Stud Alcohol* **42**, 626–641.
24. Roizen, R., Cahalan, D. and Shanks, P. (1978) Spontaneous remission among untreated problem drinkers, in *Longitudinal Research on Drug Use: Empirical Findings and Methodological Issues* (ed. D.B. Kandel), Hemisphere: Washington, DC, pp. 197–221.
25. Biernacki, P. (1986) *Pathways from Heroin Addiction: Recovery without Treatment*, Temple University Press: Philadelphia.
26. Marlatt, G.A. and Gordon, J.R. (1985) *Relapse Prevention*, Guilford Press: New York.
27. Stall, R. (1983) An examination of spontaneous remission from problem drinking in the bluegrass region of Kentucky. *J Drug Iss.* **13**, 191–206.
28. Happel, H.-V., Fischer, R. and Wittfeld, I. (1993) Selbstorganisierter Ausstieg. Überwindung der Drogenabhängigkeit ohne professionelle Hilfe (Endbericht). Integrative Drogenhilfe an der Fachhochschule Ffm L.V: Frankfurt
29. Labouvie, E. (1996) Maturing out of substance abuse: Selection and self-correction. *J Drug Iss.* **26**, 457–476.
30. Institute of Medicine. (1990) *Broadening the Base of Treatment for Alcohol Problems*, National Academy Press: Washington, DC.
31. Tuchfeld, B.S. (1976) *Changes in Patterns of Alcohol Use Without the Aid of Formal Treatment: An Exploratory Study of Former Problem Drinkers*, Research Triangle Institute: Research Triangle Park, North Carolina.
32. Mulford, H. (1988) Enhancing the natural control of drinking behavior: Catching up with common sense. *Contemp Drug Probl.* **17**, 121–334.
33. Heather, N. (1989) Psychology and brief interventions. *Br J Addict.* **84**, 357–370.
34. Heather, N. (1990) *Brief Intervention Strategies*, Pergamon: New York.
35. Heather, N. (1994) Brief interventions on the world map. *Addiction* **89**, 665–667.
36. Law, M. and Tang, J.L. (1995) An analysis of the effectiveness of interventions intended to help people stop smoking. *Arch Intern Med.* **155**(18), 1933–1941.
37. Giffen, C.A. (1991) Community intervention trial for smoking cessation (commit) – summary of design and intervention. *J Natl Cancer Inst.* **83**, 1620–1628.
38. Green, S.B., Corle, D.K., Gail. M.H. *et al.* (1995) Interplay between design and analysis for behavioral intervention trials with community as the unit of randomization. *Am J Epidemiol.* **142**(6), 587–593.

39. Hughes, J.R., Cummings, K.M. and Hyland, A. (1999) Ability of smokers to reduce their smoking and its association with future smoking cessation. *Addiction* **94**(1), 109–114.
40. Foulds, J. (1996) Strategies for smoking cessation. *Br Med Bull.* **52**, 157–173.
41. Ludwig, A.M. (1985) Cognitive processes associated with 'spontaneous' recovery from alcoholism. *J Stud Alcohol* **46**, 53–58.
42. Saunders, W.M. and Kershaw, P.W. (1979) Spontaneous remission from alcoholism: A community study. *Br J Addict.* **74**, 251–265.
43. Klingemann, H.K.-H. (1991) The motivation for change from problem alcohol and heroin use. *Br J Addict.* **86**, 727–744.
44. Sobell, L.C., Sobell, M.B., Toneatto, T. and Leo, G.I. (1993) What triggers the resolution of alcohol problems without treatment? *Alcohol: Clin Exp Res.* **17**(2), 217–224.
45. Fagerström, K.O., Kunze, M. and Schoberberger, R. (1996) Nicotine dependence versus smoking prevalence: Comparison among countries and categories of smokers. *Tob Control* **5**, 52–56.
46. Hingson, R., Scotch, N., Day, N. and Culbert, A. (1980) Recognizing and seeking help for drinking problems. *J Stud Alcohol* **11**, 1102–1117.
47. Weisner, C. (1987) The social ecology of alcohol treatment in the U.S., in *Recent Developments in Alcoholism*, Vol 5 (ed. M. Galanter), Plenum: New York, pp. 203–243.
48. Sobell, M.B. and Sobell, L.C. (1998) Guiding self-change, in *Treating Addictive Behaviors*, 2nd edition (eds W.R. Miller and N. Heather), Plenum: New York, pp. 189–202.
49. Toneatto, T., Sobell, L.C., Sobell, M.B. and Rubel, E. (1999) Natural recovery from cocaine dependence. *Psychol Addict Behav.* **13**(4), 259–268.
50. Tucker, J.A., Vuchinich, R.E. and Gladsjo, J.A. (1991) Environmental influences on relapse in substance use disorders. *Int J Addict.* **25**, 1017–1050.
51. Blomqvist, J. (1999) Treated and untreated recovery from alcohol misuse: Environmental influences and perceived reasons for change. *Subst Use Misuse* **34**(10), 1371–1406.
52. Blomqvist, J. (in press) Recovery with and without treatment. A comparison of resolutions of alcohol and drug problems. in *Thematic Meeting on the Natural History of Addictions*, 7–12 March 1999, Les Diablerets.
53. Blomqvist, J. (1999) *Inte bara behandling – vägar ut ur alkoholmissbruket*, Bokförlaget Bjurner & Bruno: Vaxholm.
54. Tucker, J.A., Vuchinich, R.E. and Pukish, M.M. (1995) Molar environmental contexts surrounding recovery by treated and untreated problem drinkers. *Exp Clin Psychopharmacol.* **3**, 195–204.
55. Tucker, J.A., Vuchinich, R.E., Gladsjo, J.A., Hawkins, J.L. and Sherrill, J.T. (1989) Environmental influences on the natural resolution of alcohol problems without treatment in *Paper Presented at a Poster Session at the Annual Meeting of the Association for the Advancement of Behavior Therapy*, November 1989, Washington, DC.
56. Tucker, J.A., Vuchinich, R.E. and Gladsjo, J.A. (1994) Environmental events surrounding natural recovery from alcohol-related problems. *J Stud Alcohol* **55**, 401–411.
57. Rumpf, H.-J., Bischof, G., Hapke, U., Meyer, C. and John, U. (2000) Studies on natural recovery from alcohol dependence: Sample selection bias by media solicitation. *Addiction* **95**, 747.
58. Vaillant, G.E. (1995) *The Natural History of Alcoholism Revisited*, Harvard University Press: Cambridge, MA.

59. Vaillant, G.E. and Milofsky, E.S. (1982) Natural history of male alcoholism. IV. Paths to recovery. *Arch Gen Psychiatry* **39**, 127–133.
60. Drew, L.R.H. (1968) Alcoholism as a self-limiting disease. *Q J Stud Alcohol* **29**, 956–967.
61. Schachter, S. (1982) Recidivism and self-cure of smoking and obesity. *Am Psychol.* **37**(4), 436–444.
62. Winick, C. (1962) Maturing out of narcotic addiction. *Bull Narc.* **14**, 1–10.
63. Carey, M.P., Snel, D.L., Carey, K.B. and Richards, C.S. (1989) Self-initiated smoking cessation: A review of the empirical literature from a stress and coping perspective. *Cognitive Ther Res.* **13**, 323–341.
64. Fiore, M.C., Novotny, T.E., Pierce, J.P. *et al.* (1990) Methods used to quit smoking in the United States. *JAMA.* **263**, 2760–2765.
65. Hughes, J.R., Fiester, S., Goldstein, M. *et al.* (1996) Practice guidelines for the treatment of patients with nicotine dependence. *Am J Psychiatry* **153**(10 Suppl.), 1–31.
66. Mariezcurrena, R. (1994) Recovery from addictions without treatment: Literature review. *Scand J Behav Ther.* **23**, 131–154.
67. Orleans, C.T., Rimer, B.K., Cristinzio, S., Keintz, M.K. and Fleisher, L. (1991) A national survey of older smokers: A treatment needs of a growning population. *Health Psychol.* **10**, 343–351.
68. U.S. Department of Health and Human Services. (1988) The health consequences of smoking: Nicotine addiction. A report of the Surgeon General. U.S. Government Printing Office: Washington, DC.
69. Jeffery, R.W. and Wing, R.R. (1983) Recidivism and self-cure of smoking and obesity: Data from population studies (Letter to the editor). *Am Psychol.* **38**, 852.
70. Rzewnicki, R. and Forgays, D.G. (1987) Recidivism and self-cure of smoking and obesity: An attempt to replicate. *Am Psychol.* **42**, 97–100.
71. Tinker, J.E. and Tucker, J.A. (1997) Motivations for weight loss and behavior change strategies associated with natural recovery from obesity. *Psychol Addict Behav.* **11**(2), 98–106.
72. Hodgins, D.C., Wynne, H. and Makarchuk, K. (1999) Pathways to recovery from gambling problems: Follow-up from a general population survey. *J Gambling Stud.* **15**, 93–104.
73. Eysenck, H.J. and Rachman, S.J. (1973) Neurosen: Ursachen und Heilmethoden: Einführung in die moderne Verhaltenstherapie (The causes and cures of neurosis). Cerlag der Wissenschaft: Berlin,-OST, Germany.
74. Finn, P. (1997) Adults recovered from stuttering without treatment: Perceptual assessment of speech normalcy. *J Speech Hear Res.* **40**, 821–831.
75. Finn, P. (1988) Recovery without treatment: A review of conceptual and methodological considerations across disciplines, in *Toward Treatment Efficacy for Stuttering: A Search for Empirical Bases* (eds A.K. Cordes and R.J. Ingham), Singular: San Diego, CA, pp. 3–25.
76. Toro, P.A. (1986) A comparison of natural and professional help. *Am J Community Psychol.* **14**, 147–159.
77. Veroff, J., Douvan, E. and Kulka, R.A. (1981) *The Inner American: A Self-Portrait From 1957–1976*, Basic: New York.
78. Rush, B. (1814) *An Inquiry Into the Effects of Ardent Spirits Upon the Human Body and Mind*, 8th edition, E. Merriam & Company: Brookfield.
79. Blomqvist, J. (1996) Paths to recovery from substance misuse: Change of lifestyle and the role of treatment. *Subst Use Misuse* **31**, 1807–1852.
80. Fillmore, K.M. (1988) *Alcohol Use Across the Life Course: A Critical Review of 70 Years of International Longitudinal Research*, Addiction Research Foundation: Toronto, Ontario.

81. Hughes, J.R., Gulliver, S.B., Fenwick, J.W. *et al.* (1992) Smoking cessation among self-quitters. *Health Psychol.* **11**, 331–334.
82. Jordon, C.M. and Oei, T.P.S. (1989) Help-seeking behaviour in problem drinkers: A review. *Br J Addict.* **84**, 979–988.
83. O'Doherty, F. and Davies, J.B. (1987) Life events and addiction: A critical review. *Br J Addict.* **82**, 127–137.
84. Smart, R.G. (1975/6) Spontaneous recovery in alcoholics: A review and analysis of the available research. *Drug Alcohol Depend.* **1**, 277–285.
85. Stall, R. and Biernacki, P. (1986) Spontaneous remission from the problematic use of substances: An inductive model derived from a comparative analysis of the alcohol, opiate, tobacco, and food/obesity literatures. *Int J Addict.* **21**, 1–23.
86. Waldorf, D. and Biernacki, P. (1982) *Natural Recovery From Heroin Addiction: A Review of the Incidence Literature*, Human Science: New York.
87. Fillmore, K.M., Hartka, E., Johnstone, B.M., Speiglman, R. and Temple, M.T. (1988) Spontaneous remission of alcohol problems: A critical review, in a paper commissioned and supported by the Institute of Medicine, June 1988, Institute of Medicine: Washington, DC.
88. Alden, L. (1988) Behavioral self-management controlled drinking strategies in a context of secondary prevention. *J Consult Clin Psychol.* **56**, 280–286.
89. Kissin, B., Rosenblatt, S.M. and Machover, K. (1968) Prognostic factors in alcoholism. *American Psychiatric Association Reports* **24**, 22–43.
90. Kendell, R.E. and Staton, M.C. (1966) The fate of untreated alcoholics. *Q J Stud Alcohol* **27**, 30–41.
91. Granfield, R. and Cloud, W. (1996) The elephant that no one sees: Natural recovery among middle-class addicts. *J Drug Iss.* **26**(1), 45–61.
92. Schasre, R. (1966) Cessation patterns among neophyte heroin users. *Int J Addict.* **1**, 23–32.
93. Snow, M. (1973) Maturing out of narcotic addiction in New York City. *Int J Addict.* **8**, 921–938.
94. Chiauzzi, E.J. and Liljegren, S. (1993) Taboo topics in addiction treatment: An empirical review of clinical folklore. *J Subst Abuse Treat.* **10**, 303–316.
95. Cunningham, J.A., Sobell, L.C. and Chow, V.M.C. (1993) What's in a label? The effects of substance types and labels on treatment considerations and stigma. *J Stud Alcohol* **54**, 693–699.
96. Cunningham, J.A., Sobell, L.C. and Sobell, M.B. (1998) Awareness of self-change as a pathway to recovery for alcohol abusers: Results from five different groups. *Addict Behav.* **23**(3), 399–404.
97. Ferris, J. (1994) Comparison of public perceptions of alcohol, drug tobacco and other addictions – moral vs. disease models, in *Paper Presented at the 20th Annual Alcohol Epidemiology Symposium*, June 1994, Ruschlikon, Switzerland.
98. Klingemann, H.K.H. (2001) Natural recovery from alcohol problems, in *International Handbook of Alcohol Dependence and Problems* (eds N. Heather, T.J. Peters and T. Stockwell), John Wiley & Sons: New York, pp. 649–662.
99. Rush, B. and Allen, B.A. (1997) Attitudes and beliefs of the general public about treatment for alcohol problems. *Can J Pub Health* **88**, 41–43.
100. Dupont, R.L. (1993) Foreword to the book 'Treating adolescent substance abuse' by G.R. Ross. Allyn and Bacon: Boston.
101. Johnson, V.E. (1980) *I'll Quit Tomorrow*, revised edition, Harper & Row: San Francisco.
102. Sack, F. (1978) Probleme der kriminalsoziologie, in *Handbuch der empirischen Sozialforschung* (Band 12, Wahlverhalten, Vorurteile, Kriminalität) (ed. R. Konig), Ferdinand Enke Verlag: Stuttgart, Germany.

103. Wagner, K. (1985) Das potential des labeling-approach: Versuch einer programmatischen neueinschätzung. *Kriminologisches J.* **4**, 267–289.
104. Hunt, M. (1998) *The New Know-Nothings: The Political Foes of the Scientific Study of Human Nature*, Transaction Publishers: Piscataway, NJ.
105. Marlatt, G.A. (1983) The controlled drinking controversy: A commentary. *Am Psychol.* **38**, 1097–1110.
106. Marlatt, G.A. (1998) *Harm Reduction: Pragmatic Strategies for Managing High-Risk Behaviors*, Guilford Press: New York.
107. Rosenberg, H. and Davis, L.A. (1994) Acceptance of moderate drinking by alcohol treatment services in the United States. *J Stud Alcohol* **55**, 167–172.
108. Sobell, M. and Sobell, L.C. (1995) Controlled drinking after 25 years: How important was the great debate? *Addiction* **90**, 1149–1153.
109. American Psychiatric Association. (1994) *Diagnostic and Statistical Manual of Mental Disorders*, 4th edition, American Psychiatric Association: Washington DC.
110. Orford, J. and Edwards, G. (1977) *Alcoholism: A Comparison of Treatment and Advice with a Study of the Influence of Marriage*, Oxford University Press: Oxford, England.
111. Vaillant, G.E. (ed.) (1980) *The Doctor's Dilemma*, 27A, CD ed. Croom Helm: London, England.
112. Emrick, C.D. (ed.) (1982) *Evaluation of Alcoholism Psychotherapy Methods*, Gardner Press: New York.
113. Miller, W.R. and Heather, N. (1986) *Treating Addictive Behaviors: Processes of Change*, Plenum: New York.
114. Sobell, L.C., Toneatto, A. and Sobell, M.B. (eds) (1990) *Behavior Therapy (Alcohol and Other Substance Abuse)*, John Wiley: New York.
115. Orford, J. (1999) Future research directions: A commentary on Project MATCH. *Addiction* **94**(1), 62–66.
116. Project MATCH Research Group. (1998) Matching alcoholism treatments to client heterogeneity: Treatment main effects and matching effects on drinking during treatment. *J Stud Alcohol* **59**(6), 631–639.
117. Project MATCH Research Group. (1998) Matching alcoholism treatments to client heterogeneity: Project MATCH three-year drinking outcomes. *Alcohol: Clin Exp Res.* **22**, 1300–1311.
118. Granfield, R. and Cloud, W. (1999) *Coming Clean: Overcoming Addiction Without Treatment*, New York University Press: New York.
119. Nathan, P.E. (1989) Treatment outcomes for alcoholism in the U.S.: Current research, in *Addictive Behaviors: Prevention and Early Intervention* (eds T. Lørberg, W.R. Miller, P.E. Nathan and G.A. Marlatt), Swets & Zeitlinger: Amsterdam, pp. 87–101.
120. Orleans, C.T., Schoenbach, V.J., Wagner, E.H. *et al.* (1991) Self-help quit smoking interventions: Effects of self-help materials, social support instructions, and telephone counseling. *J Consult Clin Psychol.* **59**, 439–448.
121. National Gambling Impact Study Commission. (1999) Final Report. Government Printing Office: Washington, DC.
122. Cunningham, J.A., Sobell, L.C., Sobell, M.B., Agrawal, S. and Toneatto, T. (1993) Barriers to treatment: Why alcohol and drug abusers delay or never seek treatment. *Addict Behav.* **18**, 347–353.
123. Cunningham, J.A., Sobell, L.C., Sobell, M.B. and Gaskin, J. (1994) Alcohol and drug abusers reasons for seeking treatment. *Addict Behav.* **19**(6), 691–696.
124. Hasin, D. and Grant, B. (1995) AA and other helpseeking for alcohol problems: Former drinkers in the U. S. general population. *J Subst Abuse* **7**, 281–292.
125. Oppenheimer, E., Sheehan, M. and Taylor, C. (1988) Letting the client speak: Drug misusers and the process of help seeking. *Br J Addict.* **83**, 635–647.

126. Smith, L. (1992) Help seeking in alcohol-dependent females. *Alcohol Alcohol* **27**, 3–9.
127. Tucker, J.A. and Davison, J.W. (2000) Waiting to see the doctor: The role of time constraints in the utlization of health and behavioral health services, in *Reframing Health Behavior Change with Behavior Economics* (eds W. Bickel and R. Vuchinich), Lawrence Erlbaum: New York, pp. 219–264.
128. Tucker, J.A. and Gladsjo, J.A. (1993) Help seeking and recovery by problem drinkers: Characteristics of drinkers who attend Alcoholics Anonymous or formal treatment or who recovered without assistance. *Addict Behav.* **18**, 529–542.
129. Gomberg, E.S.L. and Turnbull, J.E. (1990) Alcoholism in women: Pathways to treatment, in *Research Society on Alcoholism Annual Meeting*, June 1990, Toronto, Ontario, Canada.
130. Roman, P.M. (1988) Treatment issues, in *Women and Alcohol Use: A Review of the Research Literature* (ADM 88-1574) (ed. National Institute on Alcohol Abuse and Alcoholism), U.S. Government Printing Office: Washington, DC, pp. 38-45.
131. Schmidt, L. and Weisner, C. (1995) *The Emergence of Problem-Drinking Women as a Special Population in Need of Treatment*, Plenum Press: New York.
132. Schober, R. and Annis, H.M. (1996) Barriers to help-seeking for change in drinking: A gender-focused review of the literature. *Addict Behav.* **21**(1), 81–92.
133. Thom, B. (1986) Sex differences in help-seeking for alcohol problems – 1. The barriers to help-seeking. *Br J Addict.* **81**, 777–788.
134. Thom. B. (1987) Sex differences in help-seeking for alcohol problems – 2. Entry into treatment. *Br J Addict.* **82**, 989–997.
135. Weisner. C. (1993) Toward an alcohol treatment entry model: A comparison of problem drinkers in the general population and in treatment. *Alcohol: Clin Exp Res.*; **17**, 746–752.
136. Weisner, C. and Schmidt, L. (1992) Gender disparities in treatment for alcohol problems. *JAMA.* **268**, 1872–1876.
137. Beckman, L.J. and Kocel, K.M. (1982) Treatment-delivery system and alcohol abuse in women: social policy and implications. *J Soc Issues* **38**, 139–151.
138. Schmidt, L.A. and Weisner, C.M. (1999) Public health perspectives on access and need for substance abuse treatment, in *Changing Addictive Behavior: Bridging Clinical and Public Health Strategies* (eds J.A. Tucker, D.A. Donovan and G.A. Marlatt), Guilford Press: New York, pp. 67–96.
139. Duckert, F. (1989) 'Controlled drinking': A complicated and contradictory field. Nordic Council for Alcohol and Drug Research (NAD) Annankatu 29 A 23 SF-00100.
140. Blume, S.B. (1986) Women and alcohol: A review. *JAMA.* **256**, 1467–1470.
141. Klingemann, H.K.H. (1994) Environmental influences which promote or impede change in substance behaviour, in *Addiction: Processes of Change* (eds G. Edwards and M. Lader), Oxford University Press: Oxford, pp. 131–161.
142. Engemann, S. (1991) Zwei Jahre Erprobung akzeptanzorientierter, niedrigsch-wellinger Drogenarbeit im Kontaktcafé Münster. Münster: INDRO e.V.
143. National Institute on Drug Abuse. (1992) Highlights from the 1989 National Drug and Alcoholism Treatment Unit Survey (NDATUS). National Institute on Drug Abuse: Rockville, MD.
144. Sanchez-Craig, M., Spivak, K. and Davila, R. (1991) Superior outcome of females over males after brief treatment for the reduction of heavy drinking: replication and report of therapist effects. *Br J Addict.* **86**, 867–876.
145. Rounsaville, B.J. and Kleber, H.D. (1985) Untreated opiates addicts: How do they differ from those seeking treatment? *Arch Gen Psychiatry* **42**, 1072–1077.
146. Gordis, E. (1994) Alcohol and minorities. *Alcohol Alert (NIAAA)* **23**, 1–5.

147. Castro, F.G., Proescholdbell, P.J., Abeita. L. and Rodriquez, D. (1999) Ethnic and cultural minority groups, in *Addictions: A Comprehensive Guidebook* (eds B.S. McCrady and E.E. Epstein), Oxford University Press: New York, pp. 499–526.

148. Sue, S., Fujino, D.C., Hu, L., Takeuchi, T. and Zane, N.W.S. (1991) Community mental health services for ethnic minority groups: A test of the cultural responsiveness hypothesis. *J Consult Clin Psychol.* **59**, 533–540.

149. Orford, J. (1986) *Critical Conditions for Change in the Addictive Behaviors*, Plenum Press: New York.

150. Eysenck, H.J. (1952) The effects of psychotherapy: An evaluation. *J Consult Psychol.* **16**, 319–324.

151. Goldfried, M.R. (1982) *Converging Themes in Psychotherapy*, Springer: New York.

152. Janis, I.L. and Mann, L. (1968) *A Conflict-Theory Approach To Attitude Change and Decision Making*, Academic Press: New York.

153. Janis, I.L. and Mann, L. (1977) *Decision-Making: A Psychological Analysis of Conflict, Choice, and Commitment*, Free Press: New York.

154. Prochaska, J.O. and DiClemente, C.C. (1984) *The Transtheoretical Approach: Crossing Traditional Boundaries of Therapy*, Dow Jones-Irvwin: Homewood, IL.

155. Prochaska, J.O., DiClemente, C.C. and Norcross, J.C. (1992) In search of how people change. *Am Psychol.* **47**, 1102–1114.

156. Prochaska, J.O. (1983) Self-changers versus therapy versus Schachter (Letter to the editor). *Am Psychol.* **38**, 853–854.

157. Baumeister, R.F. (1996) The crystallization of discontent in the process of major life change, in *Can Personality Change?* (eds T.F. Heatherton and J.L. Weinberger), American Psychological Association: Washington, DC, pp. 281–297.

158. Ebaugh, H.R.F. (1988) *Becoming An Ex: The Process of Role Exits*, University of Chicago Press: Chicago.

159. Bandura, A. (1997) The anatomy of stages of change. *Am J Health Promot.* **12**(1), 8–10.

160. Budd, R.J. and Rollnick, S. (1996) The structure of the Readiness to Change Questionnaire: A test of Prochaska and DiClemente's transtheoretical model. *Br J Health Psychol.* **1**, 365–376.

161. Carey, K.B., Purnine, D.M., Maisto, S.A. and Carey, M.P. (1999) Assessing readiness to change substance abuse: A critical review of instruments. *Clin Psychol-Sci Pract.* **6**(3), 245–266.

162. Davidson, R. (1998) The transtheoretical model: A critical overview, in *Treating Addictive Behaviors*, 2nd edition (eds W.R. Miller and N. Heather), Plenum: New York, pp. 25–38.

163. Sutton, S. (1996) Can stages of change provide guidelines in the treatment of addictions? in *Psychotherapy, Psychological Treatments and the Addictions* (eds G. Edwards and C. Dare), Cambridge University Press: Cambridge, MA, pp. 189–205.

164. King, M.P. and Tucker, J.A. (2000) Behavior change patterns and strategies distinguishing moderation drinking and abstinence during the natural resolution of alcohol problems without treatment. *Psychol Addict Behav.* **15**, 48–55.

165. Cunningham, J.A., Ansara, D., Wild, T.C., Toneatto, T. and KoskiJannes, A. (1999) What is the price of perfection? The hidden costs of using detailed assessment instruments to measure alcohol consumption. *J Stud Alcohol* **60**(6), 756–758.

166. Gladsjo, J.A., Tucker, J.A., Hawkins, J.L. and Vuchinich, R.E. (1992) Adequacy of recall of drinking patterns and event occurrences associated with natural recovery from alcohol problems. *Addict Behav.* **17**, 347–358.

167. Klingemann, H. (1991) Coping and maintenance strategies of spontaneous remitters from problem use of alcohol and heroin in Switzerland, in *Paper*

Presented at the 17th Annual Alcohol Epidemiological Symposium, 1991, Sigtuna, Sweden.

168. Sobell, L.C., Agrawal, S. and Sobell, M.B. (1997) Factors affecting agreement between alcohol abusers' and their collaterals' reports. *J Stud Alcohol* **58**(4), 405–413.

169. Tucker, J.A. (1995) Predictors of help-seeking and the temporal relationship of help to recovery among treated and untreated recovered problem drinkers. *Addiction* **90**(6), 805–809.

170. Babor, T.F., Brown, J. and Del Boca, F.K. (1990) Validity of self-reports in applied research on addictive behaviors: Fact or fiction? *Addict Behav.* **12**, 5–32.

171. Babor, T.F., Steinberg. K., Anton. R. and DelBoca, F. (2000) Talk is cheap: Measuring drinking outcomes in clinical trials. *J Stud Alcohol* **61**(1), 55–63.

172. Maisto, S.A. and Connors, G.J. (1992) Using subject and collateral reports to measure alcohol consumption, in *Measuring Alcohol Consumption: Psychosocial and Biological Methods* (eds R.Z. Litten and J. Allen), Humana Press: Towota, NJ, pp. 73–96.

173. Maisto, S.A., McKay, J.R. and Connors, G.J. (1990) Self-report issues in substance abuse: State of the art and future directions. *Behav Assess.* **12**, 117–134.

174. Sobell, L.C., Toneatto, T. and Sobell, M.B. (1994) Behavioral assessment and treatment planning for alcohol, tobacco, and other drug problems: Current status with an emphasis on clinical applications. *Behav Ther.* **25**, 533–580.

175. De Soto, C.B., O'Donnell, W.E. and De Soto, J.L. (1989) Long-term recovery in alcoholics. *Alcohol: Clin Exp Res.* **13**, 693–697.

176. Jin, H., Rourke, S.B., Patterson, T.L., Taylor, M.J. and Grant, I. (1998) Predictors of relapse in long-term abstinent alcoholics. *J Stud Alcohol* **59**(6), 640–646.

177. Sobell, M.B., Sobell, L.C. and Kozlowksi, L.T. (1995) Dual recoveries from alcohol and smoking problems, in *Alcohol and Tobacco: From Basic Science to Clinical Practice* (NIAAA Research Monograph No 30) (eds J.B. Fertig and J.A. Allen), National Institute on Alcohol Abuse and Alcoholism: Rockville, MD, pp. 207–224.

178. Bonadonna, G. and Robustelli, G. (1988) *Handbook of Medical Oncology*, Masson: Milano, Italy.

179. Devita, V.T.J., Hellman, S. and Rosenberg, S.A. (1985) *Cancer: Principles and Practice of Oncology*, 2nd edition, J.P. Lippincott: New York.

180. Breslau, N., Peterson, E., Schultz, L., Andreski, P. and Chilcoat, H. (1996) Are smokers with alcohol disorders less likely to quit? *Am J Public Health* **86**(7), 985–990.

181. Breslin, F.C., Sobell, S.L., Sobell, L.C. and Sobell, M.B. (1997) Alcohol treatment outcome methodology: State of the art 1989–1993. *Addict Behav.* **22**(2), 145–155.

182. Heather, N. and Robertson, I. (1997) *Problem Drinking*, 3rd edition, Oxford University Press: New York.

183. Rosenberg, H. (1993) Prediction of controlled drinking by alcoholics and problem drinkers. *Psychol Bull.* **113**, 129–139.

184. Blackwell, J.S. (1983) Drifting, controlling and overcoming: Opiate users who avoid becoming chronically dependent. *J Drug Iss.* **13**, 219–235.

185. Shewan, D., Dalgarno, P., Marshall, A. *et al.* (1998) Patterns of heroin use among a non-treatment sample in Glasgow (Scotland). *Addict Res.* **6**(3), 215–234.

186. Waldorf, D. (1983) Natural recovery from opiate addiction: Some social-psychological processes of untreated recovery. *J Drug Iss.* **13**, 237–280.

187. Zinberg, N.E., Harding, W.M. and Winkeller, M. (1977) A study of social regulatory mechanism in controlled illicit drug users. *J Drug Iss.* **7**, 117–133.

188. Zinberg, N.E. and Jacobson, R.C. (1976) The natural history of 'chipping'. *Am J Psychiatry* **133**, 37–40.
189. Cohen, P. and Sas, A. (1994) Cocaine use in Amsterdam in non deviant subcultures. *Addict Res.* **2**, 71–94.
190. Hammersley, R. and Ditton, J. (1994) Cocaine careers in a sample of Scottish users. *Addict Res.* **2**, 51–70.
191. Mugford, S.K. (1995) Recreational cocaine use in three Australian cities. *Addict Res.* **3**, 95–108.
192. Waldorf, D., Reinarman, C. and Murphy, S. (1991) *Cocaine Changes: The Experience of Using and Quitting*, Temple University: Philadelphia, PA.
193. Klingemann, H.K.H. (1992) Coping and maintenance strategies of spontaneous remitters from problem use of alcohol and heroin in Switzerland. *Int J Addict.* **27**, 1359–1388.
194. Amodeo, M. and Kurtz, N. (1990) Cognitive processes and abstinence in a treated alcoholic population. *Int J Addict.* **25**, 983–1009.
195. Sobell, L.C., Cunningham, J.C., Sobell, M.B. *et al.* (1996) Fostering self-change among problem drinkers: A proactive community intervention. *Addict Behav.* **21**(6), 817–833.
196. Mann, L. (1972) Use of a 'balance sheet' procedure to improve the quality of personal decision making: A field experiment with college applicants. *J Vocat Behav.* **2**, 291–300.
197. Velicer, W.F., DiClemente, C.C., Prochaska, J.O. and Brandenburg, N. (1985) Decisional balance measure for assessing and predicting smoking status. *J Pers Soc Psychol.* **48**, 1279–1289.
198. Billings, A.G. and Moos, R.H. (1983) Psychosocial processes of recovery among alcoholics and their families: Implications for clinicians and program evaluators. *Addict Behav.* **8**, 205–218.
199. Moos, R.H., Finney, J.W. and Chan, D. (1982) The process of recovery from alcoholism. II. Comparing spouses of alcoholic patients and matched community controls. *J Stud Alcohol* **43**, 888–909.
200. Blomqvist, J. (1999) Recovery with and without treatment: A comparison of resolutions of alcohol and drug problems, in *Thematic Meeting on the Natural History of Addictions*, 7–12 March 1999, Les Diablerets.
201. Sobell, L.C., Klingemann, H., Toneatto, T., Sobell, M.B., Agrawal, S. and Leo, G.I. (in press) Cross-cultural qualitative analysis of factors associated with natural recoveries from alcohol and drug problems. *Subst Use Misuse.*

Chapter two

Self-change from alcohol and drug abuse: often cited classics

THE SETTING

As maintained by Toulmin [1], a certain event or condition can appear as a phenomenon – something that is problematic and needs explaining – only against the background of some inferred 'state of natural order'. This proposition is worth bearing in mind when revisiting and trying to summarize the key findings and major implications of some of the studies that have historically been most often cited in the debate over the existence, incidence, and character of self-change from addictive behavior. Admittedly, the selection of studies for the following brief review has by necessity been somewhat arbitrary. Nonetheless, it is evident that the vast majority of what may be termed the 'classics' in this field originated in the USA, in the 1960s and 1970s. To some extent this may be explained by the dominance, in a global perspective, of American alcohol and drug research at the time. However, the attention paid to these studies and the controversy raised by the issue of self-change may also be reflective of a cultural setting particularly conducive to making this topic stand out. Through the influence of the alcohol movement, the popular 'disease model' of drinking problems had by the early 1960s become an almost uncontested foundation for alcohol research as well as policy in the USA [2]. According to this model, alcoholism is an irreversible and inexorably progressive process, due to some inborn characteristics in certain people. Similarly, but for different reasons, narcotic drugs (i.e. at the time, opium and its derivatives) were assumed to have chemical properties making them capable of enslaving users, more or less instantly and for life. Consequently, increasing resources had been spent in the build-up of treatment facilities for people with drinking problems and in preventing any use of narcotic drugs.

Notwithstanding that such terms as 'natural recovery' or 'spontaneous remission' may initially seem compatible with a medical or biochemical notion of addiction, the suggestion that problem drinking or heroin use might be transient conditions struck at the heart of widespread and firmly rooted beliefs, and presented a challenge against strong vested interests in the prevention and treatment fields. Had social-psychological or 'natural process' models been generally accepted to account for addictive problems, the idea that many people may grow out of their problematic drinking or drug use with time would in all probability simply have stood out as 'the natural thing' [2, 3].

Before proceeding to a review of the 'classics', it should be pointed out that many of the studies that were, at the time, most frequently quoted as evidence of the existence of self-change were designed to address other research questions. Therefore, potential failures in providing a conclusive base for judgments on this specific issue should not necessarily be attributed to flaws and weaknesses in the methodology of these studies. In effect, to the extent that 'spontaneous recovery' or some semantic equivalent of that term was at all used in these studies, these terms were typically adopted as provisional metaphors for putative and still little understood, psychological or social processes.

Two tables accompany this chapter, one showing the 'classic' self-change drug studies (Table 1) and the other showing the 'classic' self-change alcohol studies (Table 2) that will be discussed. Both tables contain the following information about each study: (a) data sources; respondents; (b) principal aims; (c) main results; (d) conclusions bearing on self-change; and (e) comments.

THE 'PIONEERING STUDIES'

Charles Winick [4], often mentioned as the researcher who first drew attention to the phenomenon of self-change, conjectured that a 'maturing out' process might be partly responsible for the fact that approximately two-thirds of the 16 725 addicts (defined as regular users of opiates) originally reported to the Federal Bureau of Narcotics during 1953 and 1954 were not reported again up to the end of 1959. Based on the experience that hardly any regular narcotic user could avoid coming to the attention of the authorities during a two-year period, he argued that inactive status, with reservations for an uncertain number who had died, indicated the cessation of drug use. Winick also found that almost three-quarters of the 7234 addicts who had become inactive during the period 1955–1960 had ceased their drug use before the age of 38. In addition, a comparison of the age distribution of the inactive sample with that of the total population of addicts registered up to 1955, showed that persons aged 30–40 years were clearly over-represented in the former group. Finally, the mean length of the addiction period among the inactive cases was found to have been 8.6 years and more than 80% were found to have stopped their use before the tenth year of their addiction.

These findings led Winick to speculate about a natural 'life cycle' of heroin addiction. Essentially the hypothesis was that opiate addicts began their habit as a way of coping with the emotional challenges and strains of early adulthood and ceased with their habit when they belatedly, as the result of some homeostatic process, were able to face and cope with adult responsibilities without using drugs. As a designation of this putative process he chose the street term 'maturing out'. In a later analysis Winick [5] plotted the length of the addiction in inactive cases against age at onset. This analysis confirmed that the vast majority of the inactive cases had started their use in their late teens or early 20s and had stopped using in their late 20s or their 30s. However, a small group of persons with a very early onset proved to have been addicted for a considerably longer time than the average of the group, meaning that there was an inverse correlation between age at onset and length of addiction. Winick's conclusion was that these data essentially supported his 'maturing out' notion as regards the majority of 'intermediate users', but that long-term addicts as well as a small group of short-term users might require other designations. In retrospect, the major merit of Winick's study is that it drew attention to the fact, unrecognized or even denied at the time, that a substantial number of addict heroin users achieve enduring abstinence with time. At the same time, his calculations contain a good deal of uncertainty, lacking data for certain critical variables (e.g. mortality rates; potential treatment-effects; exact dates of cessation of drug use). Moreover, the proposed explanation did not rely on empirical data for the emotional experiences of the respondents.

A few years later, the Australian psychiatrist Les Drew [6] called attention to the fact that a large number of clinical studies showed that the quotient of identified alcoholics, in relation to the population in a specific age-group, tended to peak prior to the age of 50 years and then to decrease substantially. Drawing on the results of other studies, Drew acknowledged that one reason for the reduction of alcohol problems in older age groups might be related to increased mortality among alcohol abusers and, to a lesser degree, the beneficial effects of treatment. However, viewing these explanations as insufficient, he also found reason to conclude that a process of spontaneous recovery probably accounts for a significant proportion of alcohol abusers who cease to appear in alcohol statistics as their age increases. As potential forces involved in such a process Drew suggested a number of factors accompanying aging (e.g. increasing maturity and responsibility; decreasing drive; increasing social withdrawal; changing social pressures; and reduced financial resources). Among factors that may hamper self-change processes he included social isolation and the early onset of severe complications of alcohol abuse. As in Winick's case, what makes Drew's paper somewhat of a milestone is not that its empirical data were even close to perfection, but rather that it presented a strong and not easily ignored case against the notion of alcohol abuse as an inexorably progressive and irreversible condition, widely accepted at the time, but largely lacking an empirical basis [7].

SUBSEQUENT RESEARCH ON SELF-CHANGE

The literature pertaining to self-change published in the decades following the 'pioneering studies' presents a rather disparate mix of treatment and population studies, cross-sectional and longitudinal studies, and other addiction studies. Although varying with regard to sample size and type, overall research questions and methods, the studies to be presented in this chapter all deal with either drug or alcohol problems. Studies of self-change for gambling and cigarettes are discussed in a later chapter in this volume. The studies discussed in this chapter were selected because they were seminal studies that produced considerable controversy and public debate at the time they were published. It should be pointed out, however, that there were some early forerunners of today's research on self-change from other addictions as well. Schachter [8], in a seminal article, presented data on self-cure of smoking and obesity in two different non-therapeutic populations. In short, this study showed that about two-thirds of those who had, in a life-time perspective, tried to stop smoking or reduce their over-weight, had in fact succeeded. The successful rates of self-change in the Schachter study were higher than those usually reported for people who were treated for smoking or obesity, Schachter argues that this discrepancy may partly be due to self-selection into treatment on the part of the severest cases, but that the main explanation is likely to be that treatment studies typically report the outcome of a single attempt to quit smoking or to lose weight, whereas self-change studies reflect the cumulative effects of a life-time of efforts. Emphasizing in this way that treatment studies may give rise to flawed conclusions about the intractability of addiction problems, the author implicitly points to the need for longitudinal research on self-change as well as on the role of treatment in life-change [cf. 9].

STUDIES OF DRUG USE AND DRUG ADDICTION

Table 1 shows a variety of information on the four classic self-change drug studies that will be discussed below.

Treatment studies

Winick's study, based on official records of known drug-users, may be seen as prototypical of many of the early self-change studies in the drug field. Regrettably, studies of drug use and drug addiction in the general population are still rare [10]. As for treatment research in the drug field, a limited number of studies during the 1960s and 1970s had indicated that only a rather small percentage, seldom more than one in ten, remained continuously abstinent for periods 5–10 years after hospital treatment [11]. However, with few exceptions, these studies did not include a control group that would have permitted analyses of rates of, and forces behind, untreated recovery [12]. One of these exceptions was Burt Associates' [13] evaluation of the National Treatment Association programs, based on interviews one to three years later with 81% of 360 initially treated heroin addicts. One third of these individuals had stayed in treatment five days or less and were used as a comparison group. Almost one third (29%) were found to be 'fully recovered' (i.e. no use of illicit drugs and no arrests plus social stability during the two months prior to the interview) and an additional 37% were judged as 'partly recovered'. The crucial findings pertaining to self-change were that there were no significant differences in these respects between the treated and the control groups, and that time in treatment had no association with outcome. However, the study shows no evidence that the treatment and control groups were comparable in relevant aspects. Moreover, the two-month criterion for assessing recovery may certainly be claimed to risk confounding a temporary hiatus in one's drug use with stable recovery.

THE VIETNAM EXPERIENCE

The most frequently cited and most hotly debated self-change study in the drug field is Lee Robins' follow-up of returning Vietnam veterans, published in a series of reports and articles during the period 1973–1980. This study was originally set up by the Nixon administration through the Special Action Office on Drug Abuse Prevention to estimate the size of the drug use problem among service-men in Vietnam and after return, and to provide a basis for planning proper treatment facilities. The study employed two samples of all enlisted men who left Vietnam to return home in September 1971. The first was a simple random sample of all eligible respondents. The other was a random sample of all men who had screened 'drug positive' by urine tests before departure. Since all men were warned they would be screened, not having managed to stop using before leaving was seen as a sign of stronger addiction. After correction for a small overlap between the samples and deduction of a minority who could not be reached for an interview, the two samples comprised 451 and 469 men. The first reported analyses concerned respondents' drug use in Vietnam and during the first 8 to 12 months after their return to the US [14–17]. A later analysis was based on data from a three-year follow-up of the same samples [18]. As for drug use in Vietnam, the study found that almost half of Army enlisted men had used narcotics; 34% had tried heroin and 38% opium. Further, approximately 80% had used marijuana (not classified as narcotics in this study). Almost half of those who had used narcotics had done so more than weekly for more than six months. Overall, one out of five (20%) of all returning men admitted to having been 'addicted' to narcotics while in Vietnam (had felt 'strung out' and had experienced repeated and prolonged withdrawal symptoms). The predominant route of administration was smoking and less than 10% had ever injected. Compared with soldiers who used no drugs or only marijuana, drug users tended to be younger, and more often to be single, to be less well educated, to have been reared in broken homes and to come from larger cities. However, most of the men who used narcotic drugs in Vietnam had not done so before service and showed no signs of pre-Vietnam social deviance.

Table 1   Characteristics of classic self-change drug studies

	Author (year)			
	Winick (1962; 1964)	Snow (1973)	Burt Associates (1977)	Robins (1974 and 1993); Robins *et al.* (1974a,b; 1975; 1980)
Data sources; respondents	Official records of regular opiate users (Federal Bureau of Narcotics)	Records of drug addicts in New York (New York City Narcotics Register)	360 heroin addicts followed up for 1–3 years after treatment	Enlisted men, returning from Vietnam in September 1971
Prinicipal aims	To assess the long-term fate of registered drug users	Replication of Winick's studies, taking into account such factors as mortality and institutionalization	Evaluating the National Treatment Association's Program, by comparing treated and minimally treated subjects	To estimate drug use and problems among servicemen in Vietnam, and the need for drug addiction treatment after returning home
Main results	About 2/3 became inactive in a 5-year period. The majority stopped after <10 years use, in their late 20s or their 30s	About 1/4 stopped using in a 4-year period	Almost 1/3 had recovered (no use and social stability during 2 months before interview) and 1/3 had improved. Subjects who stayed ≤5 days did not differ from those who stayed longer	Almost half of all men had used opiates in Vietnam, and 20% had been addicted. The great majority did not resume use in the USA. Of those who did, less than 10% got re-addicted, mostly for only a brief period. Three years after return, less than 20% of those who were addicted in Vietnam had shown any signs of re-addiction

Table 1 (cont.)

	Author (year)			
	Winick (1962; 1964)	Snow (1973)	Burt Associates (1977)	Robins (1974 and 1993); Robins et al. (1974a,b; 1975; 1980)
Conclusions bearing on self-change	There may be a natural life cycle of drug addiction, and most addicts seem to 'mature out' of their addiction	'Maturing out' may be less common than suggested by Winick's studies	Many heroin addicts change for the better in a rather short time frame. Treatment does not seem to add to the recovery rate	Drug addiction is not a unitary and intractable disorder, but a complex and often transitory condition. Transitions between use, addiction and recovery are probably driven by different sets of factors
Comments	The number who actually stopped may have been exaggerated. The putative 'maturing out' process was not supported by empirical data	The lower rate of recovery may partly be explained by the unique situation in NY or by changes in the drug scene since Winick's studies	The study and control groups may not have been fully comparable. The 'recovery' criterion may have captured temporary changes	The 'Vietnam experience' may have been a facsimile of drug use and addiction in the population, demonstrating much more flux and 'natural recovery' than in treatment-seeking groups

As regards drug use during the first year after return, only about 10% of the general sample and one third of those who had tested 'drug positive' at departure proved to have used any narcotics. More interestingly, less than one in ten of all men who had used since returning had shown any signs of addiction. In the drug positive sample the corresponding proportion was one in five. That is, only 7% in the drug positive sample and 12% of all men who had been addicted in Vietnam were found to have been addicted after returning to the US [16, 17]. When the veterans were followed for an additional two-year period these figures rose somewhat. Notwithstanding, less than 20% of those who were addicted in Vietnam and had resumed narcotic use in the US were found to have been addicted at any time, and mostly for only a brief period, in the three years since returning. Collectively, these results were clearly at odds with conventional beliefs at the time. They were totally unlike reported outcomes of treated cases, which generally had shown high rates of re-addiction after as short a period as six months. Analyses of the addicted veterans' reception of treatment further showed that treatment was at best responsible for only a tiny fraction of the remarkable recovery rates. In effect, less than 2% of those who had used narcotics in Vietnam and only 6% in the 'drug positive' sample went to drug abuse treatment after returning [19]. Moreover, those who did showed the same re-addiction rates as clients in other treatment-outcome studies. Last but not least, the results indicated that recovery from drug addiction did not require abstention. Even among those who were addicted in Vietnam and had used heroin regularly after return, half of the cases were not re-addicted.

The results presented by Robins and her colleagues were met with considerable skepticism by the press as well as by large parts of the research community [20]. Indeed, attempts to dispute or explain away their findings are still emerging, even in the scientific literature. Apart from venting suspicions that the results were tailored to satisfy military authorities' interest in demonstrating that soldiers serving in Vietnam had not been consigned to a life-enduring dependence on drugs, critics have concentrated on attempts to show that the results lacked generalizability. One line of reasoning has been that the Vietnam veterans never were 'real addicts'. The argument put forth is that the strains and misery of war made addiction a 'normal reaction' and that the relatively benign outcome after return was thus irrelevant to addiction in the US. Another argument has been that the veterans' circumstances after return made them different from addicts who started their heroin use in the US (i.e. returning meant living in a new setting where one would not know where to get heroin and where factors that could serve as stimuli to relapse were essentially absent). In her 'look-back' article two decades after the initial study, Robins [20] finds reason to repudiate these objections and defend most of the original conclusions. As regards the explanation of addiction in Vietnam, she underlines that addiction had generally begun before the soldiers were exposed to combat, and that the dose-response curve, strongly indicative of a causal link, did not apply to the relation between combat exposure and addiction. Moreover, the respondents themselves did not explain their heroin use as a reaction to fear or stress, but rather as a way of making the boring life in the Army more endurable and enjoyable, factors that may explain casual use in the US as well. Since, as in 'normal' conditions, earlier anti-social behavior was indeed an important predictor of drug addiction in Vietnam, the author is inclined to see high availability and lack of alternative recreational activities as the main explanation for the remarkable rate of use, also among young men without earlier signs of personal or social problems. The argument that the impressive recovery rates after return could be explained by very limited availability and lack of stimuli to use drugs in the new environment is clearly contradicted by the fact that only a small fraction of those who continued using in the US actually became re-addicted.

According to Robins herself, looking back over the past two decades, the most important implications of the study, still not entirely incorporated in public and scientific views of heroin use, are (a) 'Few of the Vietnam addicts would have become addicted if they had remained in the US. However, their history of brief addiction followed by spontaneous recovery, both in Vietnam and afterwards, was not out of line with the American experience; only with American beliefs' (p. 1051); (b) addiction looks very different if you study it in a general population than if you study it in treated cases; and (c) addiction is a complex and many-faceted phenomenon and further understanding would be facilitated if the focus were shifted from attempts to grasp the entity of addiction to the transitions between use, addiction and recovery, most probably driven by different sets of interacting forces.

WHAT DID THE 'CLASSICS' TEACH US ABOUT DRUG ADDICTION?

On the surface, the studies just reviewed seem to indicate that recovery rates are very high among 'situational' heroin addicts, such as most of Robins' enlisted men, moderately high to high among narcotic addicts in official registers (Winick), and remarkably low among treatment-seeking addicts (cf. Maddux and Desmond). Certainly, all of the studies may be claimed to have contributed in knowledge in demonstrating that the prevailing notion of heroin as an instantly and interminably addictive drug was a myth, related to its legal status and official rhetoric rather than to empirical facts. The most probable explanation of these widely varying estimates of self-change is – besides methodological divergences – that these different types of study covered fairly different parts of the continuum of heroin use and abuse. Without reliable data allowing a comparison between studies of different drug-problem severity, it may be conjectured that heroin use and addiction among enlisted men in Vietnam may, except for the high overall prevalence, have been a fairly good representation of heroin use and addiction in the general population. Although a small proportion became re-addicted after returning, for most of these users addiction turned out to be a transient condition, strongly influenced by environmental and developmental factors. The veterans who did become re-addicted may have been more representative of a much smaller group whose problematic heroin use gets intertwined with a number of other social and psychological problems, and who eventually turn up in treatment. In this group, possibly with an earlier onset of heroin use than the average user and often with a relatively long history of problematic use before the first admission, addiction seems often to have developed into a truly self-defeating process that may be difficult to break, with or without professional help. Indeed, prevailing notions of heroin addiction as a generally progressive and irreversible condition may even function as a self-fulfilling prophecy in accelerating such a process.

As for studies of 'heroin addicts' in official registers, these may have covered a continuum ranging from users registered only for minor drug offenses to severely addicted and recurrently treated persons and this would explain the middle-range rates of self-change found in these studies. However, owing to methodological flaws in Winick's, nonetheless pioneering, study his conclusion that about two thirds of all registered addicts eventually 'mature out' of their addiction may have been somewhat exaggerated. Snow [21], in a replication based on data in the New York City Narcotics Register, tried to account for respondents who had died, been admitted to treatment or were institutionalized and found that about one fourth of the registered addicts had 'matured out' of their addiction over a four-year period. On the other hand, the lower rate found by Snow may also, at least partly, be explained by the unique situation in New York City or overall changes in the drug scene between the 1950s and the 1960s.

In their review of the incidence literature on self-change from heroin addiction Waldorf and Biernacki [22] concluded that studies over the past two decades had amply demonstrated that a significant number of heroin addicts naturally recovered from their addiction without treatment intervention. At the same time they deplored the virtual absence of studies providing information concerning the psychological, social, and environmental mechanisms and processes that may be used to bring about such changes. In addition, they pointed to the need to explore the characteristics and resources of people who recover naturally and to compare these with their treated counterparts and the larger population. With this review, and the same authors' subsequent attempt to put their proposed research program into practice [23–25], the 'second wave' of research on self-change, which provides the main focus fofthis book, may be said to have commenced, at least as regards drugs.

STUDIES OF ALCOHOLISM, DRINKING PATTERNS AND DRINKING PROBLEMS

Table 2 shows a variety of information about nine classic self-change alcohol studies, which will be discussed below.

Studies of identified alcohol abusers

Drew's [6] seminal article, building on secondary cross-sectional data, included no attempts at estimating the incidence of self-change among indivduals with alcohol problems. However, Smart [26] in the first extensive literature review in this area, reports a number of studies that followed up untreated alcohol abusers or problem drinkers at two points in time. Except for a few early studies of mostly anecdotal interest, the studies, conducted between 1965 and 1975, yielded overall recovery rates varying between 4% and 40% and annual recovery rates varying between 1% and 33%. A closer examination reveals that these differing results are most likely due to differences with regard to study groups (registered abusers, self-identified alcohol abusers in health surveys, convicted felons identified as alcohol abusers etc.), recovery criteria (not found in treatment records, abstinent, drinking without problems etc.), and follow-up periods (ranging from 6 months to 13 years).

As maintained by Smart, another problem with many of these studies is that untreated alcohol abusers may differ from those who seek and receive treatment in important respects influencing prognosis. Thus, studies of self-change should do the same as treatment studies and use control groups. However, the only two studies that had been reported at that time of self-change among treatment-seeking alcohol abusers also showed clearly different results. Thus, Kendell and Staton [27] found that half of a group of diagnosed alcohol abusers, who had been either refused or had declined treatment (Maudsley Hospital in London) and who received no treatment during the follow-up period, had improved at the follow-up 2 to 13 years later; that is, they had not experienced serious disruption due to drinking. Except for a lower proportion of abstinent cases in the untreated group, this overall improvement rate differed little from that in a treated sample from the same hospital. In contrast, Kissin, Rosenblatt, and Machover [28], in a comparative study of three different treatments, found the treated subjects to have fared much better one year after the assessment (recovery rates ranging between 17% and 20% than their untreated counterparts (only 4% improved). However, although both studies may be claimed to indicate approximately the same annual self-change rates, it is unclear whether the treated and untreated groups in any of the studies were really comparable. Thus, Kendell and Staton borrowed their treated comparison group from another study. Kissin and colleagues, on their part, tried to assign clients randomly to a waiting-list, but had to drop from their control group subjects whose request for treatment persisted beyond the six months they had been advised to wait, and who then

Table 2 Characteristics of classic studies on self-change in alcohol use

	Drew (1968)	Kendell and Staton (1966)	Kissin et al. (1968)
Data sources; respondents	Literature review of studies, reporting prevalence rates for alcoholism by age groups	Subjects who declined or were refused treatment for their alcoholism at the Maudsley Hospital, London, UK, and a comparison group of clients who were treated at the same clinic	Clients treated in three different programmes, and an untreated – waiting-list – control group
Principal aims	Assessing changes in alcoholism rates over the life-span	Assessing treatment effects and 'spontaneous recovery' in alcoholics	Comparing the outcome of different treatments and in an untreated control group
Main results	Studies from different countries display a common pattern in that the quotient of alcoholics in relation to the population in a specific age group peaks before the age of 50 and decreases substantially thereafter	Half of the untreated subjects had recovered (no serious disruption due to drinking) at the follow-up, 2–13 years after initial assessment. The improvement rate in treated subjects was similar, except for more abstinent cases	Improvement (largely abstinent and socially/ vocationally stable for 6+ months at a one-year follow-up) ranged between 17% and 20% in the treated groups, but was only 4% in the untreated groups
Conclusions bearing on self-change	The decrease of alcoholism in older age groups is not sufficiently explained by increased mortality and potential treatment effects. There may be a process of 'spontaneous recovery' driven by factors normally accompanying aging	'Spontaneous recovery' seems to be relatively common. Treatment promotes abstinence, but does not seem to add to overall improvement	'Spontaneous recovery' in alcoholism is relatively rare, and treated clients fare much better
Comments	The data used did not allow for an exact estimation of the impact of e.g. increased mortality or potential treatment effects, but the study presented a strong case against the notion of alcoholism as an inexorably progressive and irreversible 'disease'	Previous treatment experiences in the study groups were not reported. Treated and untreated samples may not have been comparable in all significant aspects	Using a waiting-list group as control may have biased results. Study attrition was almost 50%, and may have seriously jeopardized the options of making valid conclusions

Table 2 (cont.)

	Cahalan (1970); Cahalan *et al.* (1969) Knupfer (1972)	Cahalan and Room (1974)	Clark (1976); Clark and Cahalan (1976)
Data sources; respondents	National and regional probability samples of adult American citizens	National (n=1561) and regional (n=780) probability samples of adult American men	Cahalan's and Room's regional (San Francisco) sample, followed up four years after the initial interview
Principal aims	To give a detailed and representative account of American drinking practices and drinking problems	Analyzing drinking problems, their inter-correlations, and their association with drinking and with demographic and contextual factors	To assess the development over time of problem drinking and drinking problems
Main results	Drinking patterns and various drinking problems were found to be strongly associated with such factors as ethnicity, social class, sex and age. Heavy drinking and drinking problems were found to be much less prevalent in women and in the older age group. More than 3/4 of all recoveries from problematic drinking had occurred without treatment (Knupfer)	Strong ethnic and socio-economic determinants were found for both drinking and problem drinking. Specific drinking problems were found to be only modestly intercorrelated, and to vary with e.g. contextual and ecological factors. Heavy drinking and drinking problems were found to be more prevalent among men than women, and much more prevalent in younger than in older age groups	'Loss of control' as a problem-drinking symptom was found to come and go over rather brief periods (Clark). Specific symptoms showed low persistence over time, even if continued involvement with some problems was relatively common. A great proportion of all respondents with some drinking problems at Time 1 reported a complete absence of problems at Time 2
Conclusions bearing on self-change	The traditional alcoholism notion is ill fitted to capturing the general population's drinking experiences. Drinking problems tend to be transitory, generally passing with age without treatment	Problem drinking is a heterogeneous condition, and problem drinkers constitute a heterogeneous group. People may shift in and out of problem categories, depending on e.g. age and changing contextual factors	There is a great deal of flux in problem drinking. The 'key symptoms' of the alcoholism paradigm are not a one-way gate to worse problems
Comments	The studies relied on cross-sectional data and did not directly address change over time. 'Problem drinking' was predominantly assessed by a simple summary score	Analyses were mainly based on cross-sectional data, and did not directly address change over time	The follow-up period may be claimed to have been too brief to capture the prolonged course of problem drinking

Table 2 (cont.)

	Roizen et al. (1978)	Fillimore (1975, 1987a,b); Fillimore and Midanik (1984); Temple and Fillmore (1985)	Vaillant (1983, 1995)
Data sources; respondents	A subsample of 521 men in the San Francisco sample with some drinking problem at Time 1 and no treatment experience at Time 2	Probability samples, followed up over extended periods, sometimes (Fillmore, 1987b) complemented with cross-sectional analyses of various birth cohorts	Men in a community ('core city') sample, followed from adolescence until their old age. Additional data from a college sample and a follow-up of a clinical sample
Principal aims	To explore variations in the rate of 'spontaneous remission', related to initial problem severity and different outcome standards	To explore variations in drinking and drinking problems over the life-span among men and women	To explore the long-term course of alcoholism and alcohol abuse
Main results	Improvement rates varied between 11% and 71%, depending on criteria used for defining problem drinking at Time 1 and improvement at Time 2. The proportion with no problems at all at Time 2 varied between 12% (Ss scoring the highest at Time 1) and 30% (Ss scoring the lowest at Time 1)	Among men, the incidence of heavy drinking and drinking problems was found to be highest in early adulthood, decreasing with age, and chronicity of problem drinking was found to be highest in middle age. In women, heavy drinking and drinking problems were much less common in younger years, increasing slightly in the middle years, and decreasing thereafter. Chances of remission were found to vary greatly with sex and age, with the lowest rates in middle-aged men	At the age of 47, more than half of all men ever classified as alcohol abusers but never subjected to formal treatment were abstinent or drinking without symptoms. Among abusers who did receive treatment, almost half were symptom-free, of whom the majority were abstinent. Of all previous abusers drinking without symptoms at the age of 47, one-third later relapsed into alcohol abuse, as compared with less than one-fifth of those who were abstinent. Of all dependent subjects, later to have achieved abstinence for 2+ years, 4 out of 10 later relapsed, sometimes after as long as 10 years
Conclusions bearing on self-change	Since there is no natural boundary between alcoholics and non-alcoholics in the population, 'natural recovery' can be equated with a number of more or less arbitrary standards. Dealing with remission as a prognostic and a diagnostic issue requires different research designs and will yield different results	Drinking patterns and drinking problems vary with sex and age, are susceptible to cultural norms, and are often transitory. Only certain combinations of early problem drinking signs seem to predict chronicity of problems	Alcoholism has its own dynamics, and is best envisaged as a disease, in the same vein as it makes sense to regard hypertension or coronary disorder as diseases. Abstinence is the only viable alternative to addictive drinking, and the principles of AA may be said to comprise the fundamental elements of effective remedy
Comments	The study may be claimed to have had crucial implications for further research on 'natural recovery'	Controlling for potential bias due to specific historical conditions or unique aspects of specific birth cohorts did not alter overall conclusions	An alternative interpretation of the presented data is that they do show that up to half of all alcohol abusers, depending on the definition used, recover naturally, and that the 'natural course' of alcohol problems is better captured by a 'natural process' than by a disease model

had to be assigned to treatment. In addition, it should be noted that the total attrition in the study by Kissin *et al.* was almost 50%, although the rates within different samples were not reported, and that all drop-outs were classified as not improved. Thus, the reported data may well have underrated remission in the total sample as well as the difference between treated and untreated samples.

In summary, as pointed out by Blomqvist [9], making inferences about self-change from control or waiting-list groups in treatment studies may be a rather unreliable endeavor. On the one hand, because treatment effects may be cumulative, such groups should ideally include only previously untreated respondents. On the other hand, this may make them truly incomparable to treatment groups, in which re-admitted clients, probably representing the severest cases, are likely to be clearly overrepresented. Moreover, this type of study design presupposes clients voluntarily seeking treatment. However, reluctance to enter treatment may be a typical characteristic of 'self-change' and even part of the motivation to change [9].

THE 'PROBLEM DRINKING' PARADIGM

Whereas studies of treatment-seeking respondents, identified as alcohol abusers, may give a rather circumscribed picture of self-change, a quite different type of evidence, at least indirectly bearing on the same issue, comes from early survey research on drinking and drinking problems in the general population, mainly by Don Cahalan and his colleagues in the Social Research Group (later Alcohol Research Group) at Berkeley. In a forerunner to the Berkeley group's publications, Cahalan, Cisin, and Crossley [29] described the detailed drinking patterns of adult Americans, based on personal interviews with 2756 persons, representative of the total population and conducted in late 1964 and early 1965. In summary, this study showed that drinking patterns, as well as a variety of 'drinking problems' with different prevalence rates, were strongly associated with such factors as ethnic origin, social class, sex and age. The finding most relevant to the discussion of self-change was that both drinking and 'heavy drinking' were much less common among both men and women aged 50 and older than in lower age groups. Following up a subsample of the same respondents approximately 3–4 years later, Cahalan [30] more directly addressed the issue of change over time. On the basis of the heterogeneity and variability of drinking-related problems, even over rather short periods of time, found in the study, Cahalan argued that 'problem drinking', at least as a provisional concept, might better capture the realities of the general population's troubles with alcohol than the traditional notion of alcoholism. As regards self-change, this study showed that problem drinking (defined as 7+ on an 11-item problem scale) was much more common in the youngest than in older age groups. Whereas a quarter of all men aged 21–29 scored as problem drinkers, this was true for only 13% of the men aged 51–60 and only 1% of those over 70.

The prevalence of problem drinking increased with lower socio-economic status, and women showed a much lower prevalence than men. Nonetheless, the decline of problems with age was observable in all groups. Using a similar, additive problem-drinking score, Knupfer [31] examined drinking problems in two adult San Francisco probability samples (one male, and one of both sexes). Among her findings was that about one third of those who ever scored 'high' on the drinking score were stably recovered, and that less than a quarter of all recoveries had included any kind of treatment.

While these early surveys, favoring summary problems scores as the dependent variable in their analyses, came close to substituting 'drinking problems' for 'alcoholism' as a new unitary concept [32], Cahalan and Room's [33] *Problem Drinking Among American Men* adopted a disaggregated approach, entirely different from the old alcoholism paradigm. This study utilized data from the samples previously investigated by Cahalan and colleagues, supplemented by an additional, national probability sample of adult men, interviewed in 1969. The pooled data from the first two surveys yielded the total number of 1561 men aged 21 to 59, and the supplementary sample included 978 men of the same ages. In addition, the book presented some initial analyses of a probability sample of 786 San Francisco men, interviewed in late 1967 and early 1968. The core finding of this study was that problem designations seemed to be arbitrary and transitory, and that people seemed to move readily into and out of problem categories. As regards prevalence of problems, the study showed between 6% and 24% of all men to exhibit at least some sign, during the previous three years, of 1–13 types of actual or potential drinking problems. The prevalence rates of problems of 'high severity' of each type were considerably lower (often only half of that of 'minimal severity' of the same problem). Although about three-quarters of those with one problem of high severity also had at least one other problem, the overall picture was that of a very heterogeneous collection of drinking problems and people with drinking problems. Thus, even if pairwise comparisons of the problem measures showed moderately high intercorrelations, these were predominantly attributable to the large proportions of men with no problems at all. One interesting finding, for example, was that symptomatic drinking (signs of physical dependence) was more strongly associated with psychological dependence than with heavy intake. The study also confirmed earlier findings indicating strong ethnic and socio-economic determinants of drinking and drinking problems. Thus, for example, problematic drinking patterns and tangible consequences of drinking were both associated with a disadvantaged status with regard to socio-economics, ethnicity, family history, and work history. Further, this study showed the great influence of contextual or ecological factors on drinking patterns and drinking problems. For example, whereas living in an abstaining neighborhood was negatively correlated with both drinking and heavy drinking, those who did drink in this environment were more likely than others to be very heavy drinkers. At the same time, notwithstanding that heavy drinkers in dry neighborhoods did not appear to be more personally maladjusted than other heavy drinkers, the proportion experiencing tangible consequences was markedly higher. Finally, the researchers once again found heavy intake as well as problem drinking patterns to be most common in the younger age groups, declining with age.

STUDIES DIRECTLY ADDRESSING CHANGE OVER TIME

In summary, the results of the quoted studies indicated that there may be a great deal of flux in problem drinking, and that the pattern of progressive worsening of problems, suggested by the 'alcoholism' paradigm, was in many respects ill fitted to account for problem drinking in the general population. However, the analyses were based mainly on cross-sectional data and did not provide direct evidence about change over time in drinking patterns and problems. Thus, for example, they may be said to have left room for explanations of decline of drinking problems with age other than self-change (e.g. generational differences in drinking habits; increased mortality among problem drinkers; potential treatment effects). It is true that Cahalan in his 1970 book provided some longitudinal analyses; that is, using a summary index of problem drinking (based on psychological dependence and frequent intoxication) he showed that 22% of the men and 9% of the women had changed their problem-drinking status materially, in either direction, since the original interview 3–4 years earlier. In addition, both this study and the subsequent study by Cahalan and Room included some retrospective data, indicating a substantial 'maturing out' of potentially severe drinking problems.

However, it was not until Clark's [34] and Clark and Cahalan's [35] reporting of data obtained by a second wave of interviews, about four years later, of the San Francisco sample, that the Berkeley group more directly addressed the issue of change, based on repeated observations of the same respondents. In the first of these articles, Clark related 'loss of control', the core concept of the alcoholism paradigm, to other measures of heavy drinking and drinking problems. What he found was, in summary, that this variable was only one among many in predicting drinking problems, and that loss of control over drinking, instead of being a one-way gate to worse problems, appeared to come and go over even as brief a period as four years. Clark and Cahalan presented further data challenging the alleged progressiveness of alcoholism by failing to demonstrate either the persistence of 'early symptoms' of alcoholism over longer periods, or the accumulation of further drinking problems over time among respondents with such symptoms. Rather, these analyses showed that even if continued involvement in *some* alcohol problems was common, continuity of any *particular* problem over time was low. Moreover, one quarter to one half (depending on the particular problem) of all respondents with drinking problems at the time of the first interview reported a complete absence of problems four years later.

Finally, in a seminal study, based on a subsample of the same panel, Roizen, Cahalan and Shanks [36] directly addressed the question of self-change among untreated problem drinkers. The sample consisted of the 521 men who had reported some drinking problems at the time of the first interview, who never had any contact with a treatment agency or group, and who could be reached at the follow-up, about four years after the first interview. By using a variety of criteria of problem drinking at Time 1 as well as for improvement at Time 2, Roizen and colleagues found improvement rates varying from 11% to 71%. The highest rate was obtained when problem drinking was defined as 11 points on an eleven-item overall problem scale, and improvement was measured as a drop of 1+ problem score at Time 2. When the criterion was shifted to no problems at all at Time 2 (virtually no-one was totally abstinent) the recovery rate dropped to 12% in the group with the highest problem score at Time 1 and to 30% among those with the lowest score at Time 1. In a subsample of 57 men, defined to match a clinical population in problem severity, the improvement rates, depending on criteria, ranged from 14% to 59%. These findings, showing that remission can be equated with a variety of more or less arbitrary standards, falling between abstinence and any improvement, were described by the authors as a corollary of the fact that there is no natural boundary between alcohol abusers and non-alcohol abusers in the general population. In addition, they underlined that the question of remission from alcohol problems did not constitute one single research problem, but rather a number of problems, requiring different approaches. For example, they pointed out that dealing with remission as a 'prognostic' problem (i.e. following diagnosed or 'known' cases to explore factors associated with improvement and persistence) presumed the validity of the diagnostic measures that placed the respondents in the problem category in the first place. However, longitudinal studies of peoples' drinking problems can also be viewed as a way of testing various diagnostic categories, at least when these are assumed to capture a life-long condition. Indeed, the tautological claim that self-change simply represents a diagnostic failure in the first place can still be heard. By a number of analyses the authors demonstrated that designing one's study to address, for example, prognostic versus diagnostic research questions may yield different results, even when the same data are utilized.

FILLMORE'S LONGITUDINAL RESEARCH

Although the Berkeley group's panel studies demonstrated great variability in drinking and drinking problems over time, the study periods were relatively short, not allowing definite conclusions to be drawn about the long-term course of problem drinking. This limitation was partly overcome by a series of studies by Kaye Fillmore, adopting a much longer time frame. In the first study in this series Fillmore [37] followed up 206 respondents from a large study of drinking patterns and problems among 17 000 American college students, initially interviewed 20 years earlier. Although the sample size was small – the study was designed to explore the feasibility of a larger study which was subsequently not funded – the results replicated the findings of earlier cross-sectional studies by showing a substantial decrease in most types of drinking problems from early adulthood to middle age. For example, according to a summary score 42% of the men were 'problem drinkers' during their college years, but only 17% in middle age. However, the type of problems characteristic of early problem drinking did not turn out to be particularly good predictors of later problems. Rather, as the author concluded, unique combinations of early problems tended to predict unique combinations of later problems. For example, among men early drinking-related problems such as accidents, arrests, belligerence or drinking interfering with schoolwork did not predict later problems unless associated with recurrent intoxication and symptomatic drinking. Further, binge drinking tended to precede other early problems and to predict later problems, only if associated with symptomatic drinking. A noteworthy finding was that 'psycho-logical dependence' was the measure yielding the highest prevalence rates at both points in time, but had a relatively low overlap with other measures and was a poor predictor of future problem drinking. The author concludes that psychological dependence might to a certain degree be an American drinking norm, rather than a symptom of problem drinking. Another important finding emphasized by Fillmore was the tangible differences between men and women with regard to the prevalence of problem drinking as well as specific drinking problems and changes over time. Thus, for example, the decline in problem drinking with age was characteristic of men only. Actually women, with a much lower prevalence of any drinking problems during their college years, had slightly more problems in their middle age. On the basis of a closer analysis of these divergences, the author found them to indicate the influence of norms and social expectations in men's and women's drinking.

During the following years Fillmore provided further evidence of the variability over time of drinking patterns and problems in both men [38, 39] and women [40]. In a methodologically important article [41], she supplemen-ted longitudinal data with cross-sectional analyses of different birth cohorts. In this way the study was able to control for potential bias in the longitudinal analyses, due to specific historical conditions (e.g. prohibition or wartime) and other unique aspects of specific birth cohorts. Even with these controls, the study reiterated the findings that the incidence of heavy drinking, among men, was relatively high in early adulthood, decreasing with age, and that chronicity of alcohol problems (persistence over the study periods, 5–7 years) was highest in the middle years, decreasing thereafter. Reviewing evidence of spontaneous recovery from alcohol problems for a committee of the Institute of Medicine, Fillmore and colleagues [42] made the summary statement that there is:

'... a higher prevalence of problems in youth, but erratic and non-chronic with a 50–60 percent chance of remission both in the long and short term among men and more than 70 percent chance of remission among women; in middle age, a much lower prevalence, but chronic with a 30–40 percent chance of remission among men and about a 30 percent chance among women; in older age, a great deal lower prevalence of problems, which were more likely chronic, with a 60–80 percent chance of remission among men and a 50–60 percent chance of remission among women' (p. 29).

IS SELF-CHANGE PART OF THE 'NATURAL HISTORY' OF ALCOHOL PROBLEMS?

Notwithstanding that remission levels were shown to be highly responsive to measurement criteria, the Berkeley group's populations studies demonstrated a substantial amount of self-change in drinking problems, even among people with high problem-drinking scores. However, even if these studies may be claimed to have disproved the conventional picture of such problems as long-lasting, inexorably worsening with time, and even interminable, most of them obtained their data at only two points in time, often with a relatively short period of time elapsing between them. Thus, they may still be claimed not to have been able to fully refute the possibility that alcohol abusers or severe problem drinkers are strongly susceptible to relapse even after a rather long period of abstinence or problem-free drinking. This question is one of the main themes in George Vaillant's [43, 44] now 50-year-long study of the long-term course of alcohol problems, in many respects the most impressive research endeavor so far in this field, still one of those that has yielded the most varying interpretations and has caused the most heated debates. Vaillant's study is based on data from Harvard Medical School's Study of Adult Development, following a community sample of 660 men from adolescence into late middle life and further into old age. The respondents fell into two groups: an upper-middle-class College sample of 204 persons and a less privileged Core City sample of 456 persons. In his major report from 1983 Vaillant follows the 110 surviving persons in the Core City sample, ever classified as alcohol abusers (defined as 4+ points on the Problem Drinking Scale for at least one year), until the age of 47. In addition, he occasionally reports on the fate of the 26 abusers in the College sample, and some data from an eight-year follow-up of 106 persons in a clinical sample, treated in a program combining individual counseling, education on the medical aspects of alcohol use and abuse, and regular AA meetings.

As regards the origin and nature of addiction to alcohol, Vaillant [43], not totally unlike the quoted population studies, finds developing alcohol abuse to be associated with ethnic background, early social problems, and parent's alcohol problems, but not with, for example, childhood emotional problems or environmental weaknesses. Notwithstanding this, on the basis of alleged persistence of addictive drinking and the high intercorrelations between a number of measures of alcohol abuse and dependence, he maintains that alcoholism is a unitary phenomenon and is best envisaged as a disease, in the same vein as it makes sense to regard hypertension or coronary arterial disorders as diseases. In both versions of his book Vaillant further asserts that total abstinence is the only viable alternative to addictive drinking and that the principles of AA can be said to comprise all that needs to be done to achieve such a solution. However, as pointed out by Peele [45], these conclusions are not unambiguously supported by the empirical findings of Vaillant's own study. Thus, for example, more than a quarter of the untreated alcohol abusers in the Core City sample were stably abstinent at the age of 47, and almost as many were drinking without symptoms [43]. Among abusers in the same sample who had hospital or clinic visits during the follow-up period (and whose alcohol abuse was often more clearly 'progressive') slightly less than half had ceased with their abuse, predominantly by becoming abstinent. In contrast, less than one third of the clinical sample (who had been referred to AA as part of their treatment) were judged to be in stable remission at the eight-year follow-up, and only 5% had not relapsed at any time during the follow-up period [43].

To support his conclusions in the face of the above-cited findings, Vaillant, in the original edition of his book, takes the view that return to social drinking, which was a common outcome among the untreated abusers in the Core City sample, should not by necessity be equated with stable recovery. Rather, he maintains, giving a number of case histories as examples, that return to 'asymptomatic drinking' constitutes a rather ambiguous outcome, often representing borderline cases between moderate drinking and alcohol abuse. In the updated version, based on an additional 12-year follow-up [44], he presents evidence claimed to demonstrate that ex-abusers may drink for extended periods without symptoms and still relapse, and that the period of continuous abstinence required to be able to predict stable remission may in fact be much longer than the six months criterion adopted in many treatment studies. The empirical findings cited to support these claims are, e.g. that almost one third of the Core City abusers judged to be drinking socially at the age of 47 later relapsed into alcohol abuse, as compared with less than one fifth of the abstainers. Further, following up all of the 56 men in the combined Core City and College samples, ever judged to have been dependent on alcohol (DSM-III; APA, 1980) and later to have achieved abstinence for 2+ years, Vaillant finds that four out of ten relapsed at some later point in time, in some of the cases after as long as ten years or more. As regards predictors of stable abstinence he finds that neither childhood antecedents nor risk factors for alcohol abuse nor most indicators of problem severity can single out future abstainers from future chronic cases. However, becoming abstinent was moderately associated with being of Irish (as opposed to French-Mediterranean) ancestry, having ever been a binge drinker, and extensive AA involvement.

In summary, and largely in accordance with other studies, Vaillant's long-itudinal endeavor may be said to have shown that many alcohol abusers – perhaps as many as half of them, depending on how broadly abuse is defined – eventually do recover naturally, at least sometimes without quitting their drinking altogether. At the same time, his data indicate that for a smaller group the problems may develop into a more or less 'chronic' stage, from which sustained abstinence indeed seems to be the safest escape. Although admitting that alcoholism can be defined as well by a sociological as by a medical model [43], the author insists that its course in these latter cases seems to be driven by its own dynamic, legitimizing the use of the disease notion.

THE 'CLASSICS' IN THE ALCOHOL FIELD: A SUMMARY APPRAISAL

Perhaps the best way of resolving the apparent contradictions in some of Vaillant's conclusions, and of reconciling the seemingly diverging images of self-change given by studies of identified alcohol abusers and epidemiological research, is to paraphrase Room [46] , talking about 'the two worlds of alcohol problems'. Thus, from the clinical perspective addiction to alcohol may well stand out as an inexorably progressive 'disease', manifested by increasing and increasingly stereotypic drinking, accompanied by a continuous alienation from conventional life and normal social networks, and with relatively few examples of stable remission, either 'spontaneously' or by the help of treatment. In population probability samples, on the other hand, alcohol problems will typically stand out as relatively common, heterogeneous and poorly intercorre-lated, and largely transient, with self-change as the typical outcome. However, this does not necessarily mean that these two types of studies deal with groups of people who are initially and vitally different. Rather, they may be seen as focusing different parts of a continuum, the field of vision in clinical studies typically restricted to the one end, or even as using different paradigms and language to account for representations of basically the same phenomena [47]. In fact, the seemingly progressive and predictable course of alcoholism, as it appears in clinical studies, may be much of a 'retrospective illusion', created by a number of overlapping factors (e.g. that it is indeed the severest cases who tend to turn up in treatment and often to do so repeatedly; that they generally come to treatment when they are at the bottom of a cycle, and/or that people may adapt the stories they tell clinicians to what they believe to be viable in this context; cf. Peele [48]. As amply illustrated by, for example, Mulford [2], the empirical facts that some peoples' drinking tends to evolve into a vicious circle, and that the option of stable remission decreases – and is likely to require more strain – the deeper into this circle a person has come, do not prove that there are vital inborn differences between future alcohol abusers and future non-alcohol abusers.

As evidenced by this review, research and debate on self-change in the addiction field, possibly because of the perceived controversial nature of the topic, has long focused on incidence and prevalence rates. Only a few of the early studies [49–51] addressed reasons for quitting or cutting down drinking among untreated respondents. However, owing to differences in scope, methods and levels of analysis, the findings of these studies are difficult to compare and can hardly be claimed to have given a consistent picture of the forces behind self-change. What has contributed to later theorizing in the field, though, is Tuchfeld's [50] suggestion that treated and untreated recovery may be similar in form but different in content, and Vaillant's [43] attempt to discern the common 'healing forces' behind enduring solutions. At the methodological level, the study first reported by Sobell *et al.* in 1992 [52] introduced several important improvements (e.g. a thorough assessment of respondents' drinking histories to ensure that they represented recovery from severe alcohol problems; structured inventories to record environmental changes; comparisons with a non-recovered control group to avoid attributing recovery to events and experiences common to all problem drinkers). Thus setting a standard for studies to come, this study can be seen as the first in the 'second wave' of self-change research in the alcohol field.

SUMMING UP: CONCLUSIONS AND IMPLICATIONS

What can we safely deduce about self-change from these 'early classics'? In order to give a valid answer to this question, it might be helpful to turn back to the opening remarks of this chapter. The notion of self-change first attracted attention, and became the subject of dispute and controversy, at a time and place where the intended phenomenon was perceived as a challenge and a threat to widely cherished notions of alcohol and drug problems and to strong vested interests in the expanding prevention and treatment fields. At the same time, much of the empirical data that fueled the, at times, heated debate emerged as the side products of research essentially focusing on other issues. Consequently, the 'classics' can not be claimed to have given conclusive answers to simplistic questions such as 'How common is self-change?' or 'Who is the typical self-changer'? Rather, and more importantly perhaps, they may be claimed to have settled the account with a number of wide-spread, but poorly substantiated beliefs about problems related to alcohol and drug use, which at the time permeated both the popular mind and society's ways of trying to deal with these problems. In summary, they showed such problems to be multifaceted and heterogeneous, and more strongly associated with ethnic, socio-cultural, and contextual factors than with, for example, heredity or childhood experiences. As regards the long-term course of problem drinking or drug use they, contrary to what had been generally believed, demonstrated a great deal of variability and flux over often rather short periods, and a general decline of most types of problem with age. It needs to be emphasized, however, that this general picture does not refute the existence of a continuum of individual 'problem careers', ranging from temporary and relatively mild to long-lasting and increasingly severe problems, showing great resistance to any change effort, with or without treatment.

Overall, these findings fit rather poorly traditional disease or dependence paradigms, and demonstrate the need for more complex explanatory models, taking into account also psychological and sociodemographic factors as well as culturally and subculturally induced values, options, and alternatives [2, 3, 53]. As regards the incidence of self-change the early studies have amply demonstrated that people rather often change drinking and drug use habits, perceived by themselves or others to be a problem, for the better. At the same time, they have clearly indicated that recovery rates are highly sensitive to measurement (criteria used to define 'addiction' and 'improvement', study periods). Certainly, the incidence rates may also depend on how the boundary between treatment interventions and naturally occurring events and processes is drawn [9, 54].

Multiple pathways out of addiction

By demonstrating in this way that " 'spontaneous recovery' is no more a unitary phenomenon than is addiction itself" [9, p. 1819], the studies reviewed in this chapter may be claimed to have helped in pointing future research in this area to more complex, and possibly more fruitful, questions than incidence rates or allegedly stable predictors of self-change. At least indirectly, they demonstrated that there may not be one single route out of one uniform condition, defined as addiction to, for example, alcohol or heroin, but rather multiple paths out of a wide range of, more or less severe, predicaments related to substance use [53, 55]. Moreover, the options for stable recovery, as well as the specific course of the change process, may vary with problem severity as well as with personal and sociocultural circumstances. This, of course, does not make continued research any less urgent, but rather calls for more sophisticated attempts to uncover the complex web of interacting biological, psychological, social, and cultural forces that may assist people in overcoming self-defeating engagements in alcohol or drug use, whether or not this process partly occurs within the context of formal treatment. Regarded in this light, the vast implications of the studies reviewed in this chapter may be claimed to be far from having been fully acknowledged by all, either in the general public or in the research and treatment fields. Indeed, as will become evident from other chapters in this book, many of the issues raised by these early publications are still strikingly topical.

REFERENCES

1. Toulmin, S. (1961) *Foresight and Understanding*, Hutchinson: London.
2. Mulford, H.A. (1984) Rethinking the alcohol problem: A natural processes model. *J Drug Iss.* **14**, 31–43.

3. Peele, S. (1985) *The Meaning of Addiction. Compulsive Experience and Its Interpretation*, Lexington Books: Toronto.
4. Winick, C. (1962) Maturing out of narcotic addiction. *Bull Narc.* **14**, 1–10.
5. Winick, C. (1964) The life cycle of the narcotic addict and of addiction. *Bull Narc.* **16**, 1–11.
6. Drew, L.R.H. (1968) Alcoholism as a self-limiting disease. *Q J Stud Alcohol* **29**, 956–967.
7. Pattison, E.M., Sobell, M.B. and Sobell, L.C. (1977) *Emerging Concepts of Alcohol Dependence*, Springer: New York.
8. Schachter, S. (1982) Recidivism and self-cure of smoking and obesity. *Am Psychol.* **37**(4), 436–444.
9. Blomqvist, J. (1996) Paths to recovery from substance misuse: Change of lifestyle and the role of treatment. *Subst Use Misuse* **31**, 1807–1852.
10. Sobell, L.C., Ellingstad, T.P. and Sobell, M.B. (2000) Natural recovery from alcohol and drug problems: Methodological review of the research with suggestions for future directions. *Addiction* **95**, 749–769.
11. Maddux, J.F. and Desmond, D.P. (1980) New light on the maturing out hypothesis in opioid dependence. *Bull Narc.* **32**(1), 15–25.
12. Sobell, L.C., Sobell, M.B., Toneatto, T. and Leo, G.I. (1993) What triggers the resolution of alcohol problems without treatment? *Alcohol: Clin Exp Res.* **17**(2), 217–224.
13. Burt Associates. (1977) Drug Treatment in New York City and Washington DC: Follow-up Studies: NIDA.
14. Robins, L.N. (1974) *The Vietnam Drug User Returns*, U.S. Government Printing Office: Washington, D.C.
15. Robins, L.N. (1974) A follow-up sturdy of Vietnam veterans' drug use. *J Drug Iss* **4**, 61–63.
16. Robins, L.N., Davis, D.H. and Goodwin, D.W. (1974) Drug use by U.S. army enlisted men in Vietnam: A follow-up on their return home. *Am J Epidemiol.* **99**, 235–249.
17. Robins, L.N., Davis, D.H. and Nurco, D.N. (1974) How permanent was Vietnam drug addiction? *Am J Public Health Suppl.* **64**, 38–43.
18. Robins, L.N., Helzer, J.E., Hesselbrock, M. and Wish, E. (1980) Vietnam veterans three years after Vietnam: how our study changed our view of Heroin, in *Yearbook of Substance Use and Abuse* (eds L. Brill and C. Winick), Human Science Press: New York, p. 213–230.
19. Robins, L.N., Helzer, J.E. and Davis, D.H. (1975) Narcotic use in southeast Asia and afterward: An interview study of 898 Vietnam returnees. *Arch Gen Psychiatry* **32**, 955–961.
20. Robins, L.N. (1993) Vietnam veterans' rapid recovery from heroin addiction: A fluke or normal expectation? *Addiction* **88**, 1041–1054.
21. Snow, M. (1973) Maturing out of narcotic addiction in New York City. *Int J Addict.* **8**, 921–938.
22. Waldorf, D. and Biernacki, P. (1979) Natural recovery from heroin addiction: A review of the incidence literature. *J Drug Iss.* **9**(2), 282–289.
23. Waldorf, D. and Biernacki, P. (1981) The natural recovery from opiate addiction: Some preliminary findings. *J Drug Iss.* **11**, 61–74.
24. Waldorf, D. (1983) Natural recovery from opiate addiction: Some social-psychological processes of untreated recovery. *J Drug Iss.* **13**, 237–280.
25. Biernacki P. (1986) *Pathways from Heroin Addiction: Recovery without Treatment*, Temple University Press: Philadelphia.
26. Smart, R.G. (1975/76) Spontaneous recovery in alcoholics: A review and analysis of the available research. *Drug Alcohol Depend.* **1**, 277–285.

27. Kendell, R.E. and Staton, M.C. (1966) The fate of untreated alcoholics. *Q J Stud Alcohol* **27**, 30–41.
28. Kissin, B., Rosenblatt, S.M. and Machover, K. (1968) Prognostic factors in alcoholism. *Am Psychiatr Assoc Rep.* **24**, 22–43.
29. Cahalan, D., Cisin, I.H. and Crossley, H.M. (1969) *American Drinking Practices*, Rutgers Center of Alcohol Studies: New Brunswick, NJ.
30. Cahalan, D. (1970) *Problem Drinkers: A National Survey*, Jossey-Bass: San Francisco.
31. Knupfer, G. (1972) *Ex-Problem Drinkers*, University of Minnesota Press: Minneapolis.
32. Room, R. (1983) *Sociological Aspects of the Disease Concept of Alcoholism*, Plenum: New York.
33. Cahalan, D. and Room, R. (1974) *Problem Drinking Among American Men*, Rutgers Center of Alcohol Studies: New Brunswick, NJ.
34. Clark, W.B. (1976) Loss of control, heavy drinking and drinking problems in a longitudinal study. *J Stud Alcohol* **37**, 1256–1290.
35. Clark, W.B. and Cahalan, D. (1976) Changes in problem drinking over a four-year span. *Addict Behav.* **1**, 251–260.
36. Roizen, R., Cahalan, D. and Shanks, P. (1978) Spontaneous remission among untreated problem drinkers, in *Longitudinal Research on Drug Use: Empirical Findings and Methodological Issues* (ed. D.B. Kandel), Hemisphere: Washington, DC, pp. 197–221.
37. Fillmore, K.M. (1975) Relationships between specific drinking problems in early adulthood and middle age. *J Stud Alcohol* **36**, 882–907.
38. Fillmore, K.M. and Midanik, L. (1984) Chronicity of drinking problems among men: A longitudinal study. *J Stud Alcohol* **45**, 228–236.
39. Temple, M.T. and Fillmore, K.M. (1985) The variability of drinking patterns among young men, age 16–31: A longitudinal study. *Int J Addict.* **20**, 1595–1620.
40. Fillmore, K.M. (1987) Women's drinking across the adult life course as compared to men's. *Br J Addict.* **82**, 801–811.
41. Fillmore, K.M. (1987) Prevalence, incidence and chronicity of drinking patterns and problems among men as a function of age: A longitudinal and cohort analysis. *Br J Addict.* **82**, 77–83.
42. Fillmore, K.M., Hartka, E., Johnstone, B.M., Speiglman, R. and Temple, M.T. (1988) Spontaneous remission of alcohol problems: A critical review, in *Paper Commissioned and Supported by the Institute of Medicine*, 1988 June; Institute of Medicine: Washington, DC.
43. Vaillant, G.E. (1983) *The Natural History of Alcoholism: Causes, Patterns, and Paths to Recovery*, Harvard University Press: Cambridge, MA.
44. Vaillant, G.E. (1995) *The Natural History of Alcoholism Revisited*, Harvard University Press: Cambridge, MA.
45. Peele, S. (1994) *Disease or Defense?* Review of the 'Natural History of Alcoholism' by George E. Vaillant. New York Times Book Review 1983, 10.
46. Room, R. (1977) *Measurement and Distribution of Drinking Patterns and Problems in General Populations*, World Health Organization: Geneva.
47. Fillmore, K.M., Roizen, R., Kerr, W., Marvy, P., Bostrom, A. *et al.* (1999) The Changeability of Heavy Drinking: Pondering the Paradigm Shift from Chronic to Stochastic, in Paper presented at the Annual Meeting of the Kettil Bruun Society for Social and Epidemiological Research on Alcohol, May 31–June 4 1999, Montreal.
48. Peele, S. (1999) Natural remission as a natural process. Models of addiction/remission and their consequences, in *International Conference on Natural History of the Addictions*, 7–12 March 1999, Les Diablerets.

49. Saunders, W.M. and Kershaw, P.W. (1979) Spontaneous remission from alcoholism: A community study. *Br J Addict.* **74**, 251–265.
50. Tuchfeld, B.S. (1981) Spontaneous remission in alcoholics: Empirical observations and theoretical implications. *J Stud Alcohol* **42**, 626–641.
51. Ludwig, A.M. (1985) Cognitive processes associated with 'spontaneous' recovery from alcoholism. *J Stud Alcohol* **46**, 53–58.
52. Sobell, L.C., Sobell, M.B. and Toneatto, T. (1992) Recovery from alcohol problems without treatment, in *Self-control and the Addictive Behaviours* (eds N. Heather, W.R. Miller and J. Greeley), Maxwell MacMillan: New York, pp. 198–242.
53. Blomqvist, J. (1998) *Beyond Treatment? Widening the Approach to Alcohol Problems and Solutions*, Stockholm University: Stockholm
54. Moos, R. (1994) Treated or untreated, an addiction is not an island unto iself. *Addiction* **89**, 507–509.
55. Sobell, L.C, Cunningham, J.A. and Sobell, M.B. (1996) Recovery from alcohol problems with and without treatment: Prevalence in two population surveys. *Am J Public Health* **86**(7), 966–972.

Chapter three

Natural recovery or recovery without treatment from alcohol and drug problems, as seen from survey data

Much of what is known about natural recovery or self-change without treatment from alcohol and drug problems comes from general population studies or special sampling from sources other than treatment centers. In this chapter studies from large-scale population surveys and community studies as well as those from smaller samples obtained by advertising or other means will be reviewed. Such studies provide a good estimate of how many people in the larger society have alcohol and drug problems that they resolve without formal treatment. These studies also help us understand the characteristics of those who recover without treatment. The advantages and disadvantages of using various interview methods and what questions are still unanswered about natural recovery in large populations will also be examined. Practical suggestions based on this research will be further discussed in the concluding chapter of this book.

EARLY DRINKING SURVEY RESULTS

Some of the earliest interest in natural recovery began because of drinking surveys that showed declines in drinking with age. Cahalan and Room [1] found in their American Drinking Practices Survey that 25% of males aged 21–29 had high scores on a drinking problem scale. However, only 13% of those aged 50–59 and 19% over 70 had high problem scores. These results occurred for both males and females and were stronger among the higher than the lower social classes. The Cahalan and Room survey was a cross-sectional, not a longitudinal study and no estimate was made of how many people stopped drinking on their own or with active treatment. Later studies using longitudinal data have usually

65

shown that drinking practices remain stable rather than decreasing [2, 3]. Some people have argued that the difference between the longitudinal and cross-sectional studies is accounted for largely by the higher mortality of heavy drinkers, allowing only light and moderate drinkers to reach the older years [2, 4]. However, some have argued that mortality rates are an insufficient cause and natural recovery is also an important factor [5, 6].

GENERAL POPULATION SURVEY STUDIES OF SELF-CHANGE

Alcohol surveys

Several efforts have been made to determine rates of natural recovery, or recovery without treatment, in surveys of general populations. There is considerable variability in the survey methods used, the definitions of natural recovery, and how alcohol problems are defined.

The earliest survey of natural recovery used a health questionnaire at three points in the early 1960s. Bailey and Stewart [7] found that in their first survey 91 people had a current or previous drinking problem. By the second and third surveys, only 13 and six respectively were drinking within normal limits. None had psychotherapy but half had medical care related to drinking and could therefore be classed as natural recovery. This study showed a very low rate of natural recovery compared with that found in later studies. As it has a very small sample size less confidence can be had in the results.

In the early 1990s surveys of natural recovery became more numerous, larger and more sophisticated. For example, in 1995, Hasin and Grant [8] carried out the first large-scale survey of natural recovery. They used data from the National Health Interview Study conducted in 1988, which had used a well-designed sample of 43 809 people aged 18 or over in the 50 US states and the District of Columbia. They identified former drinkers, who constituted about 19% of the population. Of those former drinkers 21% were alcohol dependents and 42% were alcohol abusers, according to DSM IV criteria [9]. However, only 33% of those who were alcohol dependent and 17% who were alcohol abusers had approached Alcoholics Anonymous or sought any other kind of treatment. The majority had solved their alcohol problems without help. Many reported social pressure to cut down their drinking and this may have been sufficient to make them stop drinking.

Several important surveys of recovery without treatment have also been conducted in Canada. Sobell and her colleagues [10] used data from a national survey (*n* = 11 634) and an Ontario survey (*n* = 1034). They defined problem drinkers as those who usually drank seven or more drinks per occasion. Most of those who resolved their alcohol problems (*n* = 322 and 70) did so without using any formal treatment. The proportions for recovery without treatment were remarkably close in the two surveys (77.5% and 77.7%). However, there was a large difference in how many problem drinkers returned to moderate drinking rather than abstinence (National Survey 38%, Ontario Survey 63%). One reason suggested was that socio-economic levels and incomes are higher in Ontario than in the country as a whole and these two factors are related to the likelihood of returning to social drinking.

Recovery from addiction/dependence

Table 1 shows the provocative results of the National Longitudinal Alcohol Epidemiologic Survey (NLAES), conducted face-to-face by the U.S. Census Bureau for the National Institute on Alcohol Abuse and Alcoholism [11]. These results show that, for a large random sample of ever-alcohol-dependent Americans, remission while continuing to drink is the most typical response – especially for the large majority who are untreated. These results appear remarkable to clinicians, who are inclined to question whether those now reporting drinking without abuse or dependence (as diagnosed according to DSM-IV) could possibly have been 'alcohol dependent' (i.e. 'alcoholic' or 'addicted') in the first place or have achieved 'remission' in the second. The basis for such objections is that, indeed, natural recovery and specifically resumption of non-abusive drinking are more likely for less severely dependent alcoholics, as NLAES itself showed [11]. Nonetheless, using the standard diagnostic tool in the field, all subjects in Table 2 were diagnosable as alcohol dependent. This suggests a distinction in the minds of clinicians and others between 'diagnosed' alcoholism or dependence and 'real' alcoholics.

Table 1   National Longitudinal Alcohol Epidemiologic Survey data for past year drinking status for ever-alcohol dependent individuals[a]

Drinking outcome categories for past year	Treated individuals ($n = 223$)	Untreated individuals ($n = 3309$)
Drinking with abuse/dependence	33%	26%
Abstinent	39%	6%
Drinking without abuse/dependence	28%	58%

Adapted from [11]

Drug surveys

Not only has much less work been done on self-change from drug use, but the few published studies must be interpreted with caution. The first study [12] used the 1994 Canadian Alcohol and Drugs Survey data for over 12 000 respondents. This survey contained questions about 'ever' used drugs and 'ever' treated (i.e. 'ever gone anywhere or seen anyone for a reason that was related to [your] use of medicine or drugs?'). The wording of these questions created two problems: (1) there is no way to determine problem severity; and (2) use of treatment did not necessarily relate to drug use or serious drug problems. Also, some of the sample sizes were small, particularly for individuals treated for speed and heroin use. This study identified 'drug users' who had not used in the past year and found that very few had ever had any 'treatment', especially among regular marijuana users (16.0%), LSD users (14.1%) and cocaine/crack users (16%). Treatment rates, however, were higher for speed (20.4%) and heroin users (34.5%). Unfortunately, because of the multiple problems noted above, conclusions about self-change among drug abusers must remain uncertain.

A later provincial survey [13] examined the reasons for which 'drug users' quit. This study identified 109 former cannabis users and 26 former cocaine users who had used 50 and 10 times or more, respectively. Only 1.8% of the cannabis users and none of the cocaine users said that they quit because of treatment or as a result of advice from a physician. Most drug users mentioned factors such as growing up, personal changes, changes in responsibilities, health concerns or disappointments with the drug effects as the main reasons for stopping their use.

ESTIMATES OF RATES OF SELF-CHANGE

Table 2 shows estimated rates of self-change in the three different types of alcohol and drug studies reviewed above: (a) general population surveys; (b) community studies; and (c) snowball or media samples. All surveys or studies typically have shown that the majority of recovered respondents who reported having recovered from alcohol problems did so without treatment or self-help (e.g. Alcoholics Anonymous).

COMMUNITY STUDIES OF SELF-CHANGE

Several community-based studies of self-change from drinking problems have been conducted by a variety of approaches. In the first, Newman [14] used the records of police, treatment and social agencies and clergy to identify alcoholics in 1951. A total of 688 were found in an Ontario County and in 1961 a follow-up was made to see how many had recovered. They were deemed recovered if they did not reappear in any records at follow-up. Of the problem drinkers only 29.4% recovered without treatment as did 14.2% of alcohol addicts and 10% of chronic alcoholics. These results are far lower than would be expected from survey results. However, the criteria used were very different; people with drinking problems were not self-identified as in the surveys, but identified through records. They may have been more serious cases than those typically seen in surveys.

The community-based study of people in the Clydeside area of Scotland, by Saunders and Kershaw [15], also found a lower rate of self-change than most surveys. This survey covered 228 people who said that they 'drank too much in the past'. Some were still drinking too much; others were episodic drinkers or misclassified based on more intensive surveys. However, there were 41 past problem-drinkers, none of whom had been treated for alcoholism. Three said that advice from their GP had been important in reducing their drinking. Most had reduced their drinking because of marriage, job changes, physical illness or family advice. Of the 19 'definitely alcoholic' respondents, seven had received alcoholism treatment or had gone to Alcoholics Anonymous. The remainder, 63% or 12 cases, had recovered without treatment, but some of those seemed to have had medical advice or medical treatment for other ailments. As with the problem-drinkers, marriage, job changes and physical illness were the most important factors in recovery for the people who were 'definitely alcoholics'.

Leung and colleagues [16] conducted a 19-year follow-up of 100 people in a small Indian community. Only 46 could be re-interviewed but others ($n = 25$) were followed through medical charts or death certificates. Alcohol abuse and dependence diagnoses were made from DSM III criteria [17]. In total, 46 had stopped drinking and of those only eight, or 17%, had specific alcohol treatment. Most mentioned family pressures, and social and financial problems as the most important factors in recovery, although many could give no reason.

The community studies reviewed here give a wide range of recovery rates without treatment. It is notable, however, that the sample sizes and character-istics vary greatly, as do the criteria for alcohol problems and dependency. Also, only a few communities have been studied and they may not be representative of large populations.

SNOWBALL, MEDIA DERIVED AND CONVENIENCE SAMPLES IN SELF-CHANGE STUDIES

Numerous efforts have been made to study self-change with snowball samples, samples derived from media advertisements and other non-representative methods. Various follow-up studies, such as those by Vaillant [18], Fillmore [19] and others, established that the natural history of alcohol problems involves fluctuations over time and that some people recover with increasing age while others do not. As regards waiting-list control groups, several studies

Promoting Self-Change from Problem Substance Use

Table 2 Estimates of rates of self-change in various alcohol and drug studies

Study type	n	Type of problem drug or alcohol user	Self-change rates without treatment
General Population Surveys			
Bailey and Stewart (1967)	91	Current or previous drinking problem	13 and 6 were drinking within normal limits after 2 follow-ups
Hasin and Grant (1995)	19% of 43 809	Former drinkers	67% who were alcohol dependent and 83% of alcohol abusers recovered without treatment
Sobell et al. (1996)	11 634[a] 1034[b]	Usually drinks 7+ drinks	77.5%[a] and 77.7%[b] recovered without treatment
Cunningham et al. (1999a)	12 555	Former drug users[c]	84% of users of marijuana, 85.9% LSD, 84% crack/cocaine, 79.6% speed, 65.5% heroin were untreated
Cunningham (1999b)	109 26	Former cannabis users Former cocaine users	Only 1.8% quit because of treatment or a doctor's advice

Table 2 (cont.)

Study type	n	Type of problem drug or alcohol user	Self-change rates without treatment
Community Studies			
Newman (1965)	688	Alcoholics and problem drinkers	29.4% of problem drinkers, 14.2% of alcohol addicts and 10% of chronic alcoholics recovered without treatment
Saunders and Kershaw (1979)	228	Drinkers who drank too much in the past	No past problems, drinkers were treated; 12 of 19 definitively alcoholics were not treated
Leung et al. (1993)	46	Alcohol abusers and alcohol dependents	38 had stopped drinking without treatment
Snowball or Media Samples[d]			
Sobell et al. (1993)	120	Naturally recovered problem drinkers	99 (82.5%) abstinent without treatment; 21 (17.5%) moderate drinking without treatment
Klingemann (1991)	85	Remitted heroin cases	60% of alcohol cases and 27% of heroin cases were abstinent and treatment free
	118	Remitted alcohol cases	

[a]Canadian national sample.
[b]Ontario provincial sample.
[c]No determination made if respondent ever had a drug problem.
[d]Any reports of the snowball type do not allow for estimates of proportions of individuals recovering with treatment and are primarily qualitative studies.

found that people on waiting lists for treatment got better without treatment [20, 21], while several other studies found that waiting-list controls did not improve [22–25].

Reasons for recovery and the details of how it happens are best understood from the various studies of recovered alcoholics and alcohol abusers. Numerous studies have used people who responded from media contacts. These are not true population surveys but, rather, surveys of people who have come forward because of advertisements in newspapers, radio or TV or notice boards in strategic places. The early studies of Tuchfeld [26] and Ludwig [27] used newspaper advertisements to attract people who had recovered from alcohol problems without treatment. Tuchfeld's 51 alcoholic abusers said that they recovered mainly because of personal illness or accidents, better education about alcohol problems, religious experiences, direct interventions by friends or relatives, and financial or other problems created by alcohol. Most respondents gave more than one reason. Ludwig's questions were different and he found that his 29 people had recovered because they had hit a personal bottom, had a physical illness or a change in lifestyle, or a religious experience. A few simply lost interest in alcohol. These reasons have been reported in later studies as well.

While self-change has been a frequently reported route to recovery for cigarette smokers (estimates range from 80% to 90% of all those who stop smoking [28–33]), this phenomenon has, until recently, been largely ignored for other addictive behavior [34]. Fortunately, the last decade has witnessed increased interest in studies of self-change among substance abusers, with over half (52.6%) of all studies in a recent review published in the last eight years [34]. This same review found that 75% of the 40 studies of self-changers involved individuals with alcohol problems. The next most studied drug was heroin (22.5%). Lastly, more than half the studies (59.1%) were conducted in the United States, with 18.9% and 16.2% conducted in Europe and Canada, respectively.

Several early studies [35–37] established that there was 'maturing out' for drug addicts and that self-change occurred for alcohol, opiate, and tobacco problems. Klingemann [38] used newspapers and radio to obtain samples of recovered alcohol and heroin abusers in Switzerland. About half of the naturally recovered alcohol cases returned to social drinking but all but a few of heroin users stopped altogether. In general, the problems of both groups were the same before and after recovery. Both groups were self-conscious remitters who decided after hitting bottom or having health, financial and other problems that their addiction career should end. Klingemann showed that there are several major stages in recovery – the motivation for change, implementing this decision, and developing and maintaining a new identity. One of the largest and most comprehensive studies of alcohol problems was reported by Sobell *et al.*[39]. Using advertisements they recruited and interviewed 182 people classified as resolved abstinent, resolved non-abstinent, resolved abstinent treatment, and non-resolved (i.e. control group). To corroborate respondents' self-reports they also interviewed relatives or friends. The largest group was resolved abstinent without treatment ($n = 71$), followed by non-resolved, not treated (62). Only 28 had been treated and were abstinent. There were no differences for the resolved groups or in comparisons with the non-resolved. Most recoveries involved a cognitive appraisal of drinking pros and cons and the support of spouses. Tucker *et al.* [40] found results similar to these in their study.

Granfield and Cloud [41] also studied both alcohol and drug addicts but used a snowball sample of 46 middle-class people with stable lives, jobs and families. These people had much to lose by continuing their addictive careers; however, they were reluctant to enter treatment. Most in this study never adopted addictive lifestyles or identities and this probably helped in their recovery. Many of these findings were repeated in Burman's [42] study of 38 alcohol abusers in New Jersey obtained through the media. People who recovered eventually felt that they had too much to lose by continuing their addictive careers.

Only one study, that by Copeland [43], has focused solely on women in recovery. Copeland assembled 32 cases of women who recovered on their own, by advertisements in Sydney, Australia. Most changed because of 'concerns for current and future psychological and physical health and existential crises. A conflict developed between their impoverished lives and their self-concept as 'intelligent, middle-class women'. More than for men, these women seemed to change residences, social activities and sexual partners. However, this study had no direct comparisons with male self-changers.

WHAT CAN WE CONCLUDE ABOUT SELF-CHANGE?

When all the survey and special studies are considered together the following conclusions emerge:

- Most population surveys show that the large majority of people with alcohol problems can and do resolve them without formal treatment or self-help groups

- There are fewer relevant studies but it appears that most former illicit-drug abusers stop using drugs without formal treatment. Information about whether prescription drug users can do the same is not available yet.

- Community studies of self-change are few in number. They use different methods than the surveys. Some find the same results as the surveys and other find lower levels of self-change.

- Survey studies of self-change are larger and more useful in estimating the frequency of problems and recovery rates. However, special studies of self-selected groups are more often used to investigate the paths to recovery and the motivation for change.

- Reasons for self-change are many and varied. A recent review suggests that health and a cognitive appraisal of the pros and cons of continuing to use versus stopping are two of the more salient reasons for changing [34].

- There is some evidence from surveys that people who recover without treatment may have fewer alcohol problems (i.e. less dependent) than those who recover through treatment. While similar evidence exists for smokers [44], research in this area for drug abusers is lacking.

Clearly, studies of self-changers show that there are multiple pathways to recovery. One thing, however, is very evident from this literature and that is that self-change is the predominant pathway to recovery for alcohol and drug abusers.

CONCLUSIONS AND FUTURE DIRECTIONS: WHAT ELSE DO WE NEED TO KNOW ABOUT SELF-CHANGE?

Despite the large amount of information on self-change obtained from surveys and other studies, we lack information in several areas. As noted earlier, most studies have included only alcohol abusers. Our knowledge of self-change from illicit-drug abuse is much weaker as there are far fewer studies. Most of what we have are studies of heroin users rather than users of cocaine or marijuana, which are more popular drugs in many countries. We have no knowledge of natural recovery from prescription drug use (e.g. tranquilizers, stimulants or depressants). Further studies of illicit-drug users and prescription users are needed.

Our knowledge about self-change from alcohol problems has some serious gaps. It is not clear whether those who recover on their own from alcohol problems do so partly because their problems are less severe. We have no comparisons of the more serious health problems of those who need treatment and those who can recover without it. For example, we do not have information on rates of liver cirrhosis, hepatitis, alcohol psychoses, or other health problems in the two groups. It is not clear from the surveys whether there are some alcohol abusers whose problems are so severe that they require medical treatment and hence should not attempt to recover without treatment. Also, our studies are limited to a few countries and to only a few communities within these countries.

REFERENCES

1. Cahalan, D. and Room, R. (1974) *Problem Drinking Among American Men*, Rutgers Center of Alcohol Studies: New Brunswick, NJ.
2. Temple, M.T. and Leino, V. (1989) Long term outcomes of drinking: A 20 year longitudinal study of men. *Br J Addict.* **84**, 889–899.
3. Glynn, R.J., Bouchard, G., LoCastro, J. and Laird, N. (1985) Aging and generational effects on drinking behavior in men: Results from the Normative Aging Study. *Am J Public Health* **15**, 1413–1419.
4. Stall, R. (1987) Research issues concerning alcohol consumption among aging populations. *Drug Alcohol Depend.* **19**, 195–213.
5. Drew, L.R.H. (1968) Alcoholism as a self-limiting disease. *Q J Stud Alcohol* **29**, 956–967.
6. Harford, J.T. and Samorajski, T. (1982) Alcohol in the geriatric populations. *J Am Geriatr Soc.* **30**(1), 18–24.
7. Bailey, M.B. and Stewart, J. (1967) Normal drinking by persons reporting previous problem drinking. *Q J Stud Alcohol* **28**(2), 305–315.
8. Hasin, D. and Grant, B. (1995) AA and other help seeking for alcohol problems: Former drinkers in the U. S. general population. *J Subst Abuse* **7**, 281–292.
9. American Psychiatric Association. (1994) *Diagnostic and Statistical Manual of Mental Disorders*, 4th ed., American Psychiatric Association: Washington, D.C.
10. Sobell, L.C., Cunningham, J.A. and Sobell, M.B. (1996) Recovery from alcohol problems with and without treatment: Prevalence in two population surveys. *Am J Public Health* **86**(7), 966–972.
11. Dawson, D.A. (1996) Correlates of past-year status among treated and untreated persons with former alcohol dependence: United States, 1992. *Alcohol: Clin Exp Res.* **20**, 771–779.
12. Cunningham, J.A. (1999) Untreated remissions from drug use: The predominant pathway. *Addict Behav.* **24**(2), 267–270.
13. Cunningham, J.A., Koski-Jännes, A. and Tonneato, T. (1999) *Why do People Stop Their Drug Use? Results From a General Population Sample*. Centre for Addiction and Mental Health: Toronto, unpublished manuscript.
14. Newman, A.R. (1965) *Alcoholism in Frontenac County*, Queens University, Kingston.
15. Saunders, W.M. and Kershaw, P.W. (1979) Spontaneous remission from alcoholism: A community study. *Br J Addict.* **74**, 251–265.
16. Leung, P.K., Kinzie, J.D., Boehnlein, J.K. and Shore, J.H. (1993) A prospective study of the natural course of alcoholism in a Native American village. *J Stud Alcohol* **54**, 733–738.
17. American Psychiatric Association. (1980) *Diagnostic and Statistical Manual of Mental Disorders*, 3rd ed., American Psychiatric Association: Washington, D.C.
18. Vaillant, G.E. (1983) *The Natural History of Alcoholism: Causes, Patterns, and Paths to Recovery*, Harvard University Press: Cambridge, M.A.
19. Fillmore, K.M. (1987) Prevalence, incidence and chronicity of drinking patterns and problems among men as a function of age: A longitudinal and cohort analysis. *Br J Addict.* **82**, 77–83.
20. Kissin, B., Rosenblatt, S.M. and Machover, K. (1968) Prognostic factors in alcoholism. *Am Psychiatr Res Rep.* **24**, 22–43.
21. Kendell, R.E. and Staton, M.C. (1966) The fate of untreated alcoholics. *Q J Stud Alcohol* **27**, 30–41.
22. Alden, L. (1988) Behavioral self-management controlled drinking strategies in a context of secondary prevention. *J Consult Clin Psychol.* **56**, 280–286.

23. Barber, J.G. and Gilbertson, R. (1998) Evaluation of a self-help manual for the female partners of heavy drinkers. *Res Soc Work Pract.* **8**(2), 141–151.
24. Barber, J.G., Gilbertson, R. and Crisp, B.R. (1995) The 'pressures to change' approach to working with the partners of heavy drinkers. *Addiction* **90**, 269–276.
25. Harris, K.B. and Miller, W.R. (1990) Behavioral self-control training for problem drinkers: Components of efficacy. *Psychol Addict Behav.* **4**, 82–90.
26. Tuchfeld, B.S. (1981) Spontaneous remission in alcoholics: Empirical observations and theoretical implications. *J Stud Alcohol* **42**, 626–641.
27. Ludwig, A.M. (1985) Cognitive processes associated with 'spontaneous' recovery from alcoholism. *J Stud Alcohol* **46**, 53–58.
28. Marlatt, G.A, Curry, S. and Gordon, J.R. (1988) A longitudinal analysis of unaided smoking cessation. *J Consult Clin Psychol.* **56**, 715–720.
29. Carey, M.P., Snel, D.L., Carey, K.B. and Richards, C.S. (1989) Self-initiated smoking cessation: A review of the empirical literature from a stress and coping perspective. *Cognitive Ther Res.* **13**, 323–341.
30. Mariezcurrena, R. (1994) Recovery from addictions without treatment: Literature review. *Scand J Behav Ther.* **23**, 131–154.
31. U.S. Department of Health and Human Services. (1988) The health consequences of smoking: Nicotine addiction. A report of the Surgeon General, U.S. Government Printing Office: Washington, D.C.
32. Fiore, M.C., Novotny, T.E., Pierce, J.P. *et al.* (1990) Methods used to quit smoking in the United States. *JAMA.* **263**, 2760–2765.
33. Hughes, J.R., Fiester, S., Goldstein, M. *et al.* (1996) Practice guidelines for the treatment of patients with nicotine dependence. *Am J Psychiatry* **153**(10 Suppl.), 1–31.
34. Sobell, L.C., Ellingstad, T.P. and Sobell, M.B. (2000) Natural recovery from alcohol and drug problems: Methodological review of the research with suggestions for future directions. *Addiction* **95**, 749–769.
35. Winick, C. (1962) Maturing out of narcotic addiction. *Bull Narc.* **14**, 1–10.
36. Biernacki, P. (1986) *Pathways from Heroin Addiction: Recovery without Treatment,* Temple University Press: Philadelphia.
37. Zinberg, N.E. and Jacobson, R.C. (1976) The natural history of 'chipping'. *Am J Psychiatry* **133**, 37–40.
38. Klingemann, H.K.-H. (1991) The motivation for change from problem alcohol and heroin use. *Br J Addict.* **86**, 727–744.
39. Sobell, L.C., Sobell, M.B., Toneatto, T. and Leo, G.I. (1993) What triggers the resolution of alcohol problems without treatment? *Alcohol: Clin Exp Res.* **17**(2), 217–224.
40. Tucker, J.A., Vuchinich, R.E. and Gladsjo, J.A. (1994) Environmental events surrounding natural recovery from alcohol-related problems. *J Stud Alcohol* **55**, 401–411.
41. Granfield, R. and Cloud, W. (1996) The elephant that no one sees: Natural recovery among middle-class addicts. *J Drug Iss.* **26**(1), 45–61.
42. Burman, S. (1997) The challenge of sobriety: Natural recovery without treatment and self-help groups. *J Subst Abuse* **9**, 41–61.
43. Copeland, J. (1998) A qualitative study of self-managed change in substance dependence among women. *Contemp Drug Probl.* **25**, 321–345.
44. Fagerström, K.O., Kunze, M. and Schoberberger, R. (1996) Nicotine dependence versus smoking prevalence: Comparison among countries and categories of smokers. *Tob Control* **5**, 52–56.

Chapter four

Self-change among gamblers and cigarette smokers

This chapter reviews studies of self-change among gamblers and cigarette smokers. As will be evident, the literature is much less advanced for these types of addictive behavior than are studies of self-change from abuse of alcohol and other drugs.

GAMBLING: AN OVERVIEW

Legalized gambling has spread markedly in the United States and world-wide over the past few decades [1–3]. In the early 1900s most states had anti-gambling laws. However, starting with the initiation of state lotteries in 1964, gambling outlets have mushroomed. In the middle 1970s, 13 states had lotteries, 2 states had off-track horse-race betting, and only one state allowed casinos [4]. Today the landscape looks very different: (a) legal wagering is possible in 48 of 50 states and 90 countries worldwide; 28 states allow casino gambling; and (c) 22 states allow off-track betting [5–10]. In the USA people are spending more on legal gambling than on several other major recreational ventures (e.g. theme parks, cruise ships, recorded music, spectator sports, movies) combined [11]. Gambling and its associated problems have grown so fast and large, with legal wagering increasing from $3 billion per year in 1975 to $54 billion in 1998 [9], that the US Congress created the National Gambling Impact Study Commission (NGISC) in 1996 [9].

As might be expected, increased opportunities to gamble have resulted in an increased prevalence of gambling problems [8, 12]. It has been estimated that 7% of the population engages in a pattern of heavy, problem gambling [9]. Gambling behavior, like alcohol problems [13], appears to exist along a continuum from no problems to problem gambling to pathological gambling [12]. Pathological gambling, a diagnostic category in the DSM-IV [14], is defined as an impulse disorder with diagnostic criteria similar to those for substance dependence. In a synthesis of 119 prevalence surveys Shaffer and colleagues [3] calculated the adult lifetime and point prevalence rates for pathological gambling at 1.6% and 1.1%, respectively, while corresponding rates for problem gambling were 3.8% and 2.8%. The difference between pathological and problem gamblers is similar to the distinction in the alcohol field between severely dependent and mildly dependent (i.e. problem drinker) alcohol abusers. Gambling problems are associated with serious personal and societal consequences, particularly financial problems [8]. Like other addiction problems, gambling problems are highly comorbid with other psychological problems [8, 15].

It has been estimated that fewer than 3% of pathological gamblers have sought treatment and this number is even lower for problem gamblers [9]. In part, this is because there is a lack of treatment programs and providers for individuals with gambling problems. Consequently, because of the newness of this field, there is no established effective treatment [8] and little empirical research on the efficacy of treatment for problem gamblers [16]. Although Gamblers Anonymous (GA), which started in 1957, is the most frequently used source of help, there are also no studies of its effectiveness [8]. Lastly, with the exception of two studies [17, 18], little is known about the process of self-change from gambling. In addition, little is known about the etiology of problem gambling.

GAMBLING SURVEY RESEARCH

Because access to gambling has increased over the past two decades, epidemiological surveys of gambling involvement and gambling problems have been widely conducted throughout North America and elsewhere. Many of these surveys inquire about lifetime gambling problems as well as problems during the past year. Several surveys have found that some individuals who scored in the problem range over their lifetime reported no such problems in the past year. One interpretation of these results is that recovery has taken place. Using this criterion, a recent review of 22 North American general population surveys (median sample size of 1517 respondents) revealed mean recovery rates of 32% to 46% [12]. According to these estimates, about one-third to one-half of lifetime problem or pathological gamblers (2.2% of the adult general population) have recovered. Because treatment resources and programs have been very scarce, it is assumed that the majority of these individuals have changed on their own. Collectively, the data from these surveys suggest that, as in the surveys from the alcohol field [19], unassisted recovery from gambling is fairly common.

However, a major limitation of the self-change prevalence data is that 20 of the 22 the surveys used the South Oaks Gambling Screen (SOGS) [20] as the problem-gambling measure. Although the SOGS is widely used, information concerning its reliability and validity is limited. While it identifies problem gamblers, it appears that it may identify many people who do not acknowledge having a problem (i.e. potential false positives). For example, in one study [12] people in a general population who scored above the problem cut-off on the lifetime version of the SOGS but below the cut-off for the past year (i.e. 38% of the lifetime problem gamblers, a proportion consistent with previous surveys) were re-interviewed. It was found that, when contacted, most of these seemingly 'recovered' individuals denied ever experiencing a gambling problem and, thus, did not see themselves as recovered. The adjusted recovery rate estimated from this sample was 4.1% of the possible lifetime problem gamblers or 0.3% of the adult general population. In short, estimates of recovery rates from problem gambling based on survey data should be used carefully for the time being. Nonetheless, the results of this follow-up survey revealed that 83% of the small group of confirmed recovered gamblers had recovered without treatment. As with recovery from other addictions, resolution of gambling problems without treatment appears to be a major route to recovery.

CASE FINDING FOR NATURAL RECOVERY FROM GAMBLING

Two recent studies have investigated gambling recovery in samples recruited through the media and by word of mouth. To participate, individuals had to acknowledge a gambling problem and see themselves as no longer having a problem. Because the design of these two studies paralleled those of substance-abuse natural-recovery studies [21–24], findings from studies of different populations can be directly compared.

In one study that was conducted in Canada, a group of 43 resolved gamblers was compared with 63 active problem gamblers [17]. Of the 43 resolved, about half had had no involvement with treatment. In the other study, conducted in the USA, a group of 29 non-treated recovered gamblers were compared with 29 treated recovered gamblers [18].

A critical feature of both of these studies is the use of a non-treated control group [19]. Consequently, comparisons of treated and non-treated recoveries were possible. In both studies the treated group reported more severe gambling problems than those who changed without treatment. In other words, people with more severe problems were more likely to have sought treatment. This finding is consistent with results from alcohol studies [25, 26]. In both studies, rates of comorbid problems (e.g. depression; substance abuse problems) were very high. The majority of gamblers had suffered another disorder, and a significant number were experiencing a current disorder. Hodgins and el-Guebaly [17] did not find that comorbid problems were differentially associated with recovery through treatment, whereas Marotta [18] found that treated gamblers were more likely to have reported a history of treatment for mental disorders and substance abuse.

CHANGE PROCESSES

A major object of the two studies that used advertisements to recruit gamblers who had changed on their own was to understand the change process. In these studies reasons for change, associated life events, and factors important in maintaining the change were investigated in detail. Generally, there were few major differences between treated and non-treated gamblers. Compared with substance abusers who had changed on their own [19], naturally recovered gamblers provided a variety of reasons for quitting gambling. As expected, gamblers reported more reasons related to emotional and financial factors. No particular life events seemed to precipitate recovery. A decrease in negative life events and an increase in positive life events after they quit seemed important in maintaining the change.

Recovered Gamblers

Example 1
Did not receive any treatment since he thought he could do it on his own. Reasons for quitting were 'running out of money and having no access to any more'. Financial problems and experiencing a traumatic event also influenced his decision to quit. Specific trigger that led to stopping was 'having a bad loss at a roulette table'.

Example 2
Started gambling at 13; developed a problem in early 20s with video lottery terminals. Didn't feel he needed professional help. His reasons and actions for quitting were 'I moved back home and had things to do'. Other factors included problems with his spouse and evaluating the pros and cons of his gambling. Specific trigger that led to stopping was 'I lost a little too much at one time and that finished me.'

Compared with substance abusers who change on their own where a cognitive appraisal process has often been cited as important [22, 23, 27], gamblers were less likely to cite engaging in a 'pros and cons evaluation' as part of the decision-making process. However, in a follow-up survey 5 of 6 untreated gamblers reported that they engaged in an evaluation of the pros and cons in deciding to quit. If a cognitive evaluation is less significant in terms of affecting the change process for gamblers than for substance abusers, then a community intervention to facilitate a cognitive evaluation, as is being evaluated with alcohol abusers, may not be advisable.

MAINTAINING THE CHANGE

The naturally recovered gamblers in the two studies discussed above reported engaging in a variety of helpful actions in reaching and maintaining their goals [17, 18]. The predominant change strategies employed were behavioral and cognitive-motivational. Universally endorsed strategies included stimulus control (e.g. staying away from gambling situations) and engaging in new non-gambling activities. These results are consistent with a recent review of naturally recovered substance abusers who reported the development of nonsubstance-related interests and avoidance of substances as helpful in keeping them from relapsing [19]. Common cognitive-motivational actions included recalling past gambling-related problems, anticipating future problems, and the use of will power. These findings suggest that these strategies merit further evaluation as part of treatment and community interventions for gamblers.

Recovered Gamblers

Example 1
'I used a lot of self talk to remind myself how bad it was and how screwed up I was because of it'.

Example 2
'I don't keep a lot of money around'. 'I also avoid looking at the races in the paper'.

Example 3
Reasons for quitting were 'we moved out of the province to a spot that was not so convenient for my gambling'. Her method for quitting was 'avoiding places with machines'.

BARRIERS TO TREATMENT

In both of the natural recovery studies gamblers were asked why they did not seek treatment. The most frequently given reason was wanting to overcome the problem 'on their own'. About one-third of those in the US sample and over 80% of the Canadian sample said they wanted to change on their own. Interestingly, the same reason for delaying or not entering treatment has been reported by a great number of alcohol and drug abusers [22, 28–30].

Other frequently reported reasons for not seeking treatment were embarrassment, pride, stigma, and a perceived inability to share personal information. Again, these reasons have also been reported by naturally recovered alcohol and drug abusers [19, 22, 28–30]. One notable difference was that more than half of the gamblers in the Canadian sample reported a lack of treatment availability as a significant barrier to treatment compared with very few in the US sample.

SUMMARY OF RESULTS OF STUDIES OF GAMBLERS WHO CHANGE ON THEIR OWN

The few studies of natural recovery from gambling support the notion that there is a continuum of severity of gambling problems. At the lower end, problem gamblers are more likely than pathological gamblers to initiate and achieve change in their gambling without the use of formal treatment or self-help groups. Problem gamblers realistically believe that they can stop without an intervention. This is similar to natural recovery from alcohol problems where problem drinkers are more likely to change without treatment compared to severely dependent drinkers.

As with substance abuse, there is a need for public campaigns aimed at shifting attitudes about treatment-seeking for problem gambling. In a related regard, the results from one study using self-help materials and telephone support to promote self-change with gamblers have been reported. Problem gamblers 'who quit gambling on their own' were recruited via the media and provided with self-help materials and telephone support. At a 12-month follow-up almost 80% reported significant reduction in gambling, with over 25% reporting complete abstinence [31]. Efforts to promote self-change may be a cost-effective adjunct to formal treatment services.

Lastly, the high rate of comorbid disorders suggests that routine screening for comorbid problems is important. In recognition of the high rate of comorbid substance abuse and mental health problems, it may be helpful to integrate or coordinate gambling interventions with general mental health and addiction services. Certainly, parallel training of service providers is warranted.

AN OVERVIEW OF THE SMOKING FIELD

The fact that 'tobacco smoking accounts for more morbidity and mortality in the US today than use of all other psychoactive drugs combined' [32] attests to its costs and consequences. Cigarette smoking is the leading cause of cancer [33] and is a significant risk factor for cardiovascular disease (i.e. up to 30% of all deaths due to cardiovascular disease are a result of smoking cigarettes [34]).

Another factor that contributes to the enormousness of the problem of cigarette smoking is the sheer numbers of individuals who smoke cigarettes.

Although a recent US survey revealed that in the month prior to the interview twice as many 12-year-old individuals reported using alcohol as those who reported smoking cigarettes (65% vs. 32% [35]), the fact remains that there is no level of cigarette smoking that is without risk whereas low levels of alcohol consumption appear to have a health protective effect [36, 37]. Put differently, all current smokers can be considered as having problems with nicotine or as at risk of developing problems compared with a reported 10% to 15% of those who consume alcohol [38–40].

In contrast to other addictive behavior, studies reporting smoking cessation without treatment have been the rule rather than the exception [41–43]. These studies show that natural recovery or self-change is a common route to recovery for cigarette smokers, with estimates ranging from 80% to 90% of all those who stop smoking doing so on their own [33, 42, 44–48]. One reason that the prevalence of quitting cigarettes on one's own is high compared with treatment recovery is that treatment programs for smoking have not been prevalent and third party (e.g. insurance) reimbursement for treatment has been virtually nonexistent [46, 49, 50].

Public health campaigns and brief interventions have also been widely used to promote smoking cessation [51–56]. Such interventions, designed to encourage smokers to quit mainly on their own with a minimal level of assistance, are very cost-effective [57]. The Community Intervention Trial (COMMIT) for smoking cessation is an excellent example of a community-based proactive effort to reach smokers through existing social institutions [51, 58, 59]. The primary intervention, designed to work through communities, uses media channels, major organizations, and social institutions capable of influencing smoking behavior in large groups of individuals. Lastly, smokers who have stopped on their own tend to be less dependent on nicotine than smokers who seek help [60]. These results are similar to those in the alcohol field [26, 61] and parallel the studies of natural recovery from gambling reviewed earlier. Two questions will be addressed in this section. First, how frequent is natural recovery from smoking, and, second, what are the factors leading to quitting smoking cigarettes?

NICOTINE SURVEY RESEARCH

While 'smoking is the leading cause of preventable morbidity and mortality in the United States, and the health benefits of quitting smoking are substantial,' [62, p. 657], about a quarter of all adults continue to smoke cigarettes [63, 64]. Accompanying declining smoking prevalence rates has been a corresponding increase in smoking cessation rates. Table 1 shows the prevalence of smoking cessation (quit rates) for adults 18 years of age and older in the United States over a 30-year period.

Although smoking cessation rates have doubled (24% in 1965 to 49% in

Table 1   Percentage of ever smokers 18 years and older who quit smoking cigarettes, United States, 1965–1995

Variable	Year									
	1965	1970	1974	1979	1983	1988	1992	1993	1994	1995
Overall	24	33	35	39	40	46	47	50	49	49
By sex										
Male	28	37	39	43	45	49	50	52	51	51
Female	19	27	28	33	35	42	43	47	46	46
By age (years)										
18–24	13	19	20	23	21	27	19	22	21	25
25–44	21	30	29	33	34	37	37	39	38	38
45–64	28	36	40	44	46	53	54	57	57	55
≥65	46	57	57	63	65	70	73	76	77	75

[1]National Health Interview Surveys, selected years.
Source: http://www.cdc.gov/nccdphp/osh/tab_3.htm (accessed 2.9.1999)

1995) over the past 30 years, smoking rates are increasing for some groups (e.g. college students; certain ethnic groups).For substance abusers and individuals with other clinical disorders smoking rates are very high. The fact that 50% to 80% of individuals with substance use and mental health problems smoke cigarettes [64, 65] attests to the fact that these problems are highly comorbid with smoking.

Another possibility for estimating cessation rates is observations of control groups in randomized controlled trials. In this regard, a meta-analysis of 633 smoking cessation studies reported an annual cessation rate of 6% for the control groups [66].

There are several limitations of survey data. First, the definitions of smoking have varied between the surveys. Second, because smoking is associated with considerable morbidity and mortality, differential mortality can introduce substantial bias into the estimates. Third, population-based studies often miss a substantial part of disadvantaged people, drop-outs, illiterate and institutionalized individuals, and others who might have substantially higher rates of addictive behavior. Survey data, however, are more representative of the entire population than are trials with recruited volunteers.

Although cross-sectional data are the best source to estimate prevalence in populations, longitudinal studies are more helpful for identifying factors related to recovery. In one such study, a representative sample of adolescents enrolled in 1971 in New York State public secondary high schools at ages 15 to 16 was repeatedly interviewed over 19 years [67]. This study looked at the natural history of all drug use, including smoking, from adolescence to the mid-thirties. There was no initiation into cigarettes after age 29. Among the 80% of men who reported that they had ever tried cigarettes, 53% still smoked cigarettes in the past year in 1990, when they were 34–35 years old. Among women, 78% tried cigarettes, and 48% of those were still smoking at 34–35 years. Monthly cigarette consumption peaked from age 19 to age 22 at 48% of the total cohort. Thereafter, over 12 years it decreased slightly but constantly to 36%. This represents a cessation rate of 2% per year. Of all drugs, alcohol and cigarettes showed the most persistence in consumption. With respect to quantities consumed, cigarette smoking appeared to be the most stable form of drug behavior.

A nationally representative cohort of the US population was taken from the First National Health and Nutrition Examination Survey 1971–1975 and the NHANES I Epidemiologic Follow-up Survey 1982–1984. The baseline survey found 36% to be current smokers. At a follow-up conducted a mean of 9.2 years after the initial survey, 21% had quit for at least one year prior to the follow-up. Significant factors in predicting quitting were: (1) older age; (2) white race; (3) fewer cigarettes smoked per day; (4) higher household income; and (5) hospitalization in the follow-up period [68].

Sorlie and Kannel [69] used life-table methods to describe the cumulative rates of cigarette smoking cessation or resumption in the cohort in the Framingham Study. At 22 years after the start of the study, probability of smoking cessation among those smoking cigarettes at entry was 68% for men and 53% for women. Cumulative probability curves were almost linear. Men, older participants, and those who smoked less at entry had higher cessation rates than participants with opposite characteristics. The heavier smokers had a lower cessation rate but were also less likely to resume smoking if they had quit. Thus, they appeared to have been more successful at maintaining their nonsmoking state.

THE PROCESS UNDERLYING NATURAL RECOVERY FROM SMOKING

Although smoking is the most prevalent health-risk behavior of the beginning of the 21st century and 80% to 90% of smokers who stop do so on their own [33, 42], very little is known about the qualitative aspects of the cessation process (i.e. how they accomplished cessation; what was associated with either the process of stopping or the maintenance of quitting). Klingemann [70], in a recent review, found some limited evidence for a cognitive build-up of motivation as a preparatory strategy for quitting smoking as well as contradictory results for the role of social support for maintaining the change. The overwhelming reason for quitting smoking, however, has been health-related concern [71, 72].

Several longitudinal studies have reported psychological or psychosocial predictors of smoking cessation. For example, a longitudinal study that analysed the unaided smoking cessation attempts of 153 smokers who were intending to quit at New Year's day found socio-demographic factors, amount of smoking, use of strategies, and motivation to quit to be associated with abstinence at a two-year follow-up [48]. In addition, variables related to short-term outcome were generally unrelated to long-term outcome.

The Normative Aging Study used newspaper advertisements to recruit smokers intending to quit [43]. Predictors of smoking relapse among self-quitters included shorter periods of abstinence on prior quit attempts, greater pre-cessation consumption of alcoholic beverages, and lower pre-cessation levels of confidence in quitting.

In a review of smoking cessation relapse and maintenance factors, Ockene and her colleagues [73] evaluated 11 prospective studies of 'self-quitters'. Predictors of long-term cessation (i.e. 6 months) by self-quitters were (a) more education; (b) more confidence in ability to not relapse; (c) fewer cigarettes smoked; (d) less alcohol use; (e) higher confidence and self-efficacy; and (f) less social pressure to smoke.

CONCLUDING COMMENTS AND FUTURE RESEARCH NEEDS FOR SMOKING AND GAMBLING PROBLEMS

For both gambling and cigarette smoking there is clear evidence that self-change is a viable and documented experience. For smoking there is a long established literature showing that self-change is the predominant pathway to change. What is notably lacking, however, are studies probing the qualitative self-change process for smokers. Although published studies for gamblers are infrequent, early surveys suggest that self-change is also a major pathway to recovery from gambling problems. In addition, the results from the few studies of gamblers who have changed on their own have found that reasons for changing, maintenance factors and barriers to treatment entry are very similar to those found for natural recovery from alcohol and drug abuse.

As the prevalence of gambling problems has grown there is a parallel need to develop effective and appealing interventions as well as a need to understand the recovery process. Because gambling encompasses various forms of addictive behavior (e.g. video poker machines, slot machines, casino games, horse racing, sports betting, bingo), an interesting challenge for the field will be to compare gambling problems and recovery as a function of type of gambling involvement (e.g. casino games versus day trading).

In North America, the characteristics of smokers have changed over the past decade. Today smoking is inversely related to education and income level. Thus, smoking cessation strategies once effective for middle-class white male smokers may not be effective for today's smokers. Further, it has been suggested that social contextual factors such as stress and living environment need to be explored further as they may be relevant to long-term smoking cessation. As with gambling, there is a serious lack of studies that have examined the qualitative nature of the change process.

REFERENCES

1. Becona, E. (1996) Prevalence surveys of problem and pathological gambling in Europe: The cases of Germany, Holland and Spain. *J Gambling Stud.* **12**, 179–192.
2. Dickerson, M.G., Baron, E., Hong, S.-M. and Cottrell, D. (1996) Estimating the extent and degree of gambling related problems in the Australian Population: A national survey. *J Gambling Stud.* **12**, 161–178.
3. Shaffer, H.J., Hall, M.N. and Vander Bilt, K.J. (1999) Estimating the prevalence of disordered gambling behavior in the United States and Canada: A research synthesis. *Am J Public Health* **89**, 1369–1376.
4. Commission on the Review of the National Policy Towards Gambling. (1976) Gambling in America. Washington, DC.
5. Ladouceur, R. (1996) The prevalence of pathological gambling in Canada. *J Gambling Stud.* **12**(2), 129–142.
6. Lamberton, A. and Oei, T.P.S. (1997) Problem gambling in adults: An overview. *Clin Psychol Rev.* **4**(2), 84–104.
7. Lesieur, H. and Rosenthal, R.J. (1991) Pathological gambling: A review of the literature (Prepared for the American Psychiatric Association Task Force on DSM-IV Committee on Disorders of Impulse Control, not elsewhere classified). *J Gambling Stud.* **7**, 5–39.
8. López Viets, V.C.L. (1998) Treating pathological gambling, in *Treating Addictive Behaviors*, 2nd edn (eds W.R. Miller and N. Heather), Plenum: New York, pp. 259–270.
9. National Gambling Impact Study Commission. (1999) Final Report. Government Printing Office: Washington, DC.
10. Petry, N.M. and Bickel, W.K. (1999) Therapeutic alliance and psychiatric severity as predictors of completion of treatment for opioid dependence. *Psychiatr Serv.* **50**(2), 219–227.
11. Christiansen, E.M. (1999) The United States 1998 gross annual wager: Steady growth study. *Int Gaming Wagering Business* **20**, 17, 22–25.
12. Hodgins, D.C., Wynne, H. and Makarchuk, K. (1999) Pathways to recovery from gambling problems: Follow-up from a general population survey. *J Gambling Stud.* **15**, 93–104.
13. Sobell, M.B. and Sobell, L.C. (1993) Treatment for problem drinkers: A public health priority, in *Addictive Behaviors Across the Lifespan: Prevention, Treatment, and Policy Issues* (eds J.S. Baer, G.A. Marlatt and R.J. McMahon), Sage: Beverly Hills, CA, pp. 138–157.
14. American Psychiatric Association. (1994) *Diagnostic and Statistical Manual of Mental Disorders*, 4th edn. American Psychiatric Association: Washington, DC.
15. Crockford, D. and El-Guebaly, N. (1998) Psychiatric comorbidity in pathological gambling. A critical review. *Can J Psychiatry* **43**, 43–50.
16. Petry, N.M. and Armentano, C. (1999) Prevalence, assessment, and treatment of pathological gambling: A review. *Psychiatr Serv.* **50**(8), 1021–1027.
17. Hodgins, D.C. and El-Guebaly, N. (2000) Natural and treatment-assisted recovery from gambling problems: A comparison of resolved and active gamblers. *Addiction* **95**, 777–789.

18. Marotta, J.J. (1999) Recovery from gambling with and without treatment (Unpublished dissertation, University of Nevada).
19. Sobell, L.C., Ellingstad, T.P. and Sobell, M.B. (2000) Natural recovery from alcohol and drug problems: Methodological review of the research with suggestions for future directions. *Addiction* **95**, 749–769.
20. Lesieur, H. and Blume, S. (1987) The South Oaks Gambling Screen (SOGS): A new instrument for the identification of pathological gamblers. *Am J Psychiatry* **144**, 1184–1188.
21. Klingemann, H. (1991) Coping and maintenance strategies of spontaneous remitters from problem use of alcohol and heroin in Switzerland, in *Paper Presented at the 17th Annual Alcohol Epidemiological Symposium*, Sigtuna, Sweden.
22. Sobell, L.C., Sobell, M.B., Toneatto, T. and Leo, G.I. (1993) What triggers the resolution of alcohol problems without treatment? *Alcohol: Clin Exp Res.* **17**(2), 217–224.
23. Toneatto, T., Sobell, L.C., Sobell, M.B. and Rubel, E. (1999) Natural recovery from cocaine dependence. *Psychol Addict Behav.* **13**(4), 259–268.
24. Tucker, J.A., Vuchinich, R.E. and Gladsjo, J.A. (1994) Environmental events surrounding natural recovery from alcohol-related problems. *J Stud Alcohol* **55**, 401–411.
25. Humphreys, K., Moos, R.H. and Cohen, C. (1997) Social and community resources and long-term recovery from treated and untreated alcoholism. *J Stud Alcohol* **58**(3), 231–238.
26. Sobell LC, Cunningham JA, Sobell MB. (1996) Recovery from alcohol problems with and without treatment: Prevalence in two population surveys. *Am J Public Health* **86**(7), 966–972.
27. Sobell, L.C., Klingemann, H., Toneatto, T., Sobell, M.B., Agrawal, S. and Leo, G.I. (2001) Alcohol and drug abusers' perceived reasons for self-change in Canada and Switzerland: Computer assisted content analysis. *Subst Use Misuse* **34**.
28. Cunningham, J.A., Sobell, L.C., Sobell, M.B., Agrawal, S. and Toneatto, T. (1993) Barriers to treatment: Why alcohol and drug abusers delay or never seek treatment. *Addict Behav.* **18**, 347–353.
29. Hingson, R., Mangione, T., Meyers, A. and Scotch, N. (1982) Seeking help for drinking problems: A study in the Boston metropolitan area. *J Stud Alcohol* **43**, 273–288.
30. Thom, B. (1986) Sex differences in help-seeking for alcohol problems. 1. The barriers to help-seeking. *Br J Addict.* **81**, 777–788.
31. Hodgins, D. (in press) Motivational enhancement and self-help treatments for problem gambling. *J Consult Clin Psychol.*
32. Brady, K. (ed.) (1995) *Prevalence, Consequences and Costs of Tobacco, Drug and Alcohol Use in the United States*, Josiah Macy Jr. Foundation: New York.
33. US Department of Health and Human Services. (1988) The health consequences of smoking: nicotine addiction. A report of the Surgeon General. US Government Printing Office: Washington, DC.
34. US Department of Health and Human Services. (1990) The health benefits of smoking cessation. A report of the Surgeon General. US Government Printing Office: Washington, DC.
35. Substance Abuse and Mental Health Administration. (1997) National Household Survey on Drug Abuse: Main findings 1995. US Department of Health and Human Services: Rockville, MD.
36. Bondy, S.J., Rehm, J., Ashley, M.J., Walsh, G., Single, E. and Room, R. (1999) Low-risk drinking guidelines: The scientific evidence. *Can J Public Health* **90**(4), 264–270.

37. Thakker, K.D. (1998) An overview of health risks and benefits of alcohol consumption. *Alcohol: Clin Exp Res.* **22**(7), 285S–298S.
38. Substance Abuse and Mental Health Administration. (1997) A guide to substance abuse services for primary care clinicians (Treatment Improvement Protocol Series, No. 24). US Department of Health and Human Services: Rockville, MD.
39. Substance Abuse and Mental Health Administration. (1997) National Household Survey on Drug Abuse: Population estimates 1996. US Department of Health and Human Services: Rockville, MD.
40. Substance Abuse and Mental Health Administration. (1998) National Household Survey on Drug Abuse: Main findings1996. US Department of Health and Human Services: Rockville, MD.
41. Davis, A.L., Faust, R. and Ordentlich, M. (1984) Self-help smoking cessation and maintenance programs: A comparative study with 12-month follow-up by the American Lung Association. *Am J Public Health* **74**, 1212–1217.
42. Fiore, M.C., Novotny, T.E., Pierce, J.P. *et al.* (1990) Methods used to quit smoking in the United States. *JAMA.* **263**, 2760–2765.
43. Garvey, A.J., Bliss, R.E., Hitchcock, J.L., Heinold, J.W. and Rosner, B. (1992) Predictors of smoking relapse among self-quitters: A report from the normative aging study. *Addict Behav.* **17**, 367–377.
44. Carey, M.P., Snel, D.L., Carey, K.B. and Richards, C.S. (1989) Self-initiated smoking cessation: A review of the empirical literature from a stress and coping perspective. *Cognitive Ther Res.* **13**, 323–341.
45. Ershoff, D.H., Quinn, V.P. and Mullen, P.D. (1995) Relapse prevention among women who stop smoking early in pregnancy: A randomized clinical trial of a self-help intervention. *Am J Prev Med.* **11**, 178–184.
46. Hughes. J.R., Fiester, S., Goldstein, M. *et al.* (1996) Practice guidelines for the treatment of patients with nicotine dependence. *Am J Psychiatry* **153**(10), 1–31.
47. Mariezcurrena, R. (1994) Recovery from addictions without treatment: Literature review. *Scand J Behav Ther.* **23**, 131–154.
48. Marlatt, G.A., Curry, S. and Gordon, J.R. (1988) A longitudinal analysis of unaided smoking cessation. *J Consult Clin Psychol.* **56**, 715–720.
49. Law, M. and Tang, J.L. (1995) An analysis of the effectiveness of interventions intended to help people stop smoking. *Arch Intern Med.* **155**(18), 1933–1941.
50. McClure, J.B., Skaar, K., Tsoh, J., Wetter, D.W., Cinciripini, P.M. and Gritz, E.R. (1997) Smoking cessation. 3. Needed health care policy changes. *Behav Med.* **23**(1), 29–34.
51. Hughes, J.R., Cummings, K.M. and Hyland, A. (1999) Ability of smokers to reduce their smoking and its association with future smoking cessation. *Addiction* **94**(1), 109–114.
52. Lando, H.A., Hellerstedt, W.L., Pirie, P.L. and McGovern, P.G. (1992) Brief supportive telephone outreach as a recruitment and intervention strategy for smoking cessation. *Am J Public Health* **82**, 41–46.
53. Orleans, C.T., Schoenbach, V.J., Wagner, E.H. *et al.* (1991) Self-help quit smoking interventions: Effects of self-help materials, social support instructions, and telephone counseling. *J Consult Clin Psychol.* **59**, 439–448.
54. Richmond, R.L. (1996) Retracing the steps of Marco Polo: From clinical trials to diffusion of interventions for smokers. *Addict Behav.* **21**(6), 683–697.
55. Rollnick, S., Butler, C.C. and Stott, N. (1997) Helping smokers make decisions: The enhancement of brief interventions for general medical practice. *Patient Educ Couns.* **31**, 191–203.
56. Skaar, K.L., Tsoh, J.Y., McClure, J.B. *et al.* (1997) Smoking cessation. 1. An overview of research. *Behav Med.* **23**(1), 5–13.
57. Foulds, J. (1996) Strategies for smoking cessation. *Br Med Bull.* **52**, 157–173.

58. Giffen, C.A. (1991) Community intervention trial for smoking cessation (commit) – summary of design and intervention. *J Natl Cancer Inst.* **83**, 1620–1628.
59. Green, S.B., Corle, D.K., Gail, M.H. *et al.* (1995) Interplay between design and analysis for behavioral intervention trials with community as the unit of randomization. *Am J Epidemiol.* **142**(6), 587–593.
60. Fagerström, K.O., Kunze, M. and Schoberberger, R. (1996) Nicotine dependence versus smoking prevalence: Comparison among countries and categories of smokers. *Tob Control* **5**, 52–56.
61. Sobell, L.C., Sobell, M.B. and Toneatto, T. (eds). (1992) Recovery from alcohol problems without treatment, in *Self-Control and the Addictive Behaviours* (eds N. Heather, W.R. Miller and J. Greeley), Maxwell MacMillan: New York, pp. 198–242.
62. Wetter, D.W., Fiore, M.C., Gritz, E.R. *et al.* (1998) The agency for health care policy and research: Smoking cessation clinical practice guidelines: Findings and implications. *American Psychologist* **53**, 657–669.
63. Emery, S., Gilpin, E.A., Ake, C., Farkas, A.J. and Pierce, J.P. (2000) Characterizing and identifying 'Hard-Core' smokers: Implications for further reducing smoking prevalence. *Am J Public Health* **90**, 387–394.
64. Hurt, R.D., Offord, K.P., Croghan, I.T. *et al.* (1996) Mortality following inpatient addictions treatment: Role of tobacco use in a community-based cohort. *JAMA.* **275**(14), 1097–1103.
65. Hughes, J.R., Hatsukami, D.K., Mitchell, J.E. and Dahlgren, L.A. (1986) Prevalence of smoking among psychiatric outpatients. *Am J Psychiatry* **143**, 993–997.
66. Viswesvaran, C. and Schmidt, F.L. (1992) A meta-analytic comparison of the effectiveness of smoking cessation methods. *J Appl Psychol.* **77**, 554–561.
67. Chen, K. and Kandel, D.B. (1995) The natural history of drug use from adolescence to the mid-thirties in a general population sample. *Am J Public Health* **85**, 41–47.
68. McWorther, W.P., Boyd, G.M. and Mattson, M.E. (1990) Predictors of quitting smoking: the NHANES I follow-up experience. *J Clin Epidemiol.* **43**, 1399–1405.
69. Sorlie, P.D. and Kannel, W.B. (1990) A description of cigarette smoking cessation and resumption in the Framingham Study. *Prev Med.* **19**, 335–345.
70. Klingemann, H.K.H. (1994) Environmental influences which promote or impede change in substance behaviour, in *Addiction: Processes of Change* (eds G. Edwards and M. Lader), Oxford University Press, Oxford, pp. 131–161.
71. Curry, S.J., Grothaus, L. and McBride, C. (1997) Reasons for quitting: Intrinsic and extrinsic motivation for smoking cessation in a population-based sample of smokers. *Addict Behav.* **22**(6), 727–739.
72. Freund, K.M., Dagostino, R.B., Belanger, A.J., Kannel, W.B. and Stokes, J. (1992) Predictors of smoking cessation: The Framingham study. *Am J Epidemiol.* **135**, 957–964.
73. Ockene, J.K., Emmons, K.M., Mermelstein, R.J. *et al.* (2000) Relapse and maintenance issues for smoking cessation. *Health Psychol.* **19**, 17–31.

Chapter five

Hostile and favorable societal climates for self-change: some lessons for policy makers

INTRODUCTION

Voting behavior, fashion wear, eating habits, exercise, and hygiene: we do not live in a societal limbo; rather our actions are influenced and affected by societal values, trends, commercials and campaigns. From our daily experience it seems plausible that social and cognitive processes go hand in hand. In the area of natural-recovery research, decisional processes of self-change are often seen as occurring within the individual or from interactions between individuals rather than from societal forces. This is not surprising, given the influence of clinical psychology and psychiatry as well as the methodological difficulties involved in measuring the impact of society on individual behavior.

From a sociological point of view, the role of secondary groups, weak ties, and the societal climate, all of which may promote or impede self-change, has been largely neglected. Exceptions are the concept of 'social capital', including multi-level resources for change [1, p. 137–138, see also Chapter 9 in this book] and recent attempts to apply staging models to understanding health behavior and lifestyle changes within an organizational and environmental framework [2]. As a result of this restricted point of view, our understanding of the self-change process will suffer from an individualistic (vs. societal) bias and will remain incomplete. To address this gap, this chapter sets out to show links between the individual clinical view and social factors such as 'public images of addiction', 'treatment systems', 'the role of the media' and 'policy measures', as macro-societal aspects that are of interest to policy makers.

IMAGES OF ALCOHOL AND DRUG ADDICTION IN THE GENERAL
POPULATION: STIGMA OR SOCIAL SUPPORT?

Societal beliefs about social problems and their nature will shape individual and
collective responses to individual self-change. How visible are these problems?
How confident are we that people may eventually change their eating disorders,
heroin or alcohol use, or pathological gambling on their own? How much time
should we reasonably give them?

The answers to these questions will depend on the overall concept of
addiction or the paradigms that prevail in societies. Is addictive behavior seen
as a medical problem, a social problem or as criminal or immoral in nature? The
disease concept 'once an addict always an addict' is at the heart of natural-
recovery research. Of interest in this context is the informal social response to
natural recovery! It can be assumed that the social support potential quitters
experience in their attempt at self-change will be contingent upon the images in
the general population and more precisely in the quitters' reference groups.

The preceding point can be illustrated with an example from Switzerland.
Consecutive surveys on 'The image of the alcoholic in the mirror of the public
opinion', conducted in 1975, 1984 and 1992, demonstrated highly visible
alcohol problems and a highly sensitized population. For example, 28% of the
respondents in 1975 knew of a case of alcoholism; in 1984 the figure was 40%
[3, p. 28], and remained at a relatively high level in 1992. During the same
period (1975 to 1992) known cases, especially at the workplace, rose from 6% to
15% [4, p. 594–595]. Interestingly, the characteristics that society attributes to
'alcoholics' have remained relatively unchanged and, in fact, are consistent with
the traditional disease concept and moral connotations of addiction.

More specifically, as compared with the earlier studies, the 1992 survey
showed that respondents were less inclined to attribute the characteristics 'lazy',
'stubborn', and 'egoistic' when confronted with a semantic profile of the typical
alcoholic. While a more medical view could be hailed as reduced stigma, there
can be a downside to de-stigmatization. For example, although an individual is
seen as suffering from a disorder rather than 'misbehaving', the perception of
severely dependent alcohol abusers as 'chronically diseased' and plagued with
'loss of control' may reduce access to occupations that may require a great
degree of control over machinery and may discourage social support for such
careers among substance abusers. Klingemann's study on alcohol and heroin
remitters has shown how much these images are still at work, even when the
respondents have achieved change. Successful heroin self-changers experienced
negative reactions by others far more frequently than alcohol spontaneous
remitters, which again points to differences in stigmatization as a function of
societal images [5, p. 1376–1378]. For potential self-changers who are in the
pre-contemplation phase or weighing strategies for implementing change, the
images of the nature of addiction and the public visibility of successful natural
recovery are very important, as reflected in a Canadian survey. Whereas 53% of

the respondents who had overcome their dependence without treatment knew of similar cases, only 14% in a general population group were aware of self-change cases. The other groups (significant others of self-changers, unsuccessful self-changers and treatment cases) fell within these two extremes. Societal stigma kept people from telling others about their successful self-change process: only 5% of self-changers said they did not tell others that they had stopped smoking, whereas five times more (24%) did not tell others they had stopped drinking [6, p. 401]. The foregoing discussion of the social climate for self-change clearly shows that it occurs and, more importantly, that there is a need to promote environmental conditions favorable for natural recovery.

TREATMENT SYSTEM AND TREATMENT OPTIONS – LUCKY TO BE A HEROIN USER?

Self-change or natural recovery is defined as the successful resolution of a behavior perceived as problematic, a process which is primarily driven by the motivation and power of the individual and social forces, without reliance on treatment or expert help or intervention. The chances that an individual changes through self-change rather than treatment will depend to some extent on the availability of treatment resources [7]. This availability will vary greatly according to the type of problem at a given time.

The treatment of smoking illustrates this point nicely. Hughes claims that the statement '90–95% of smokers who quit, quit on their own without treatment' is no longer correct given the increasing sale of medications such as over-the-counter nicotine replacements and bupropion in the United States; therefore 37% of all quits in 1998 could be attributed to medication use. He draws an interesting parallel between the growth of this branch of the treatment industry with the response to some psychiatric disorders: 'Few clinicians . . . thought of depression as a disorder at the time. Most believed it could be cured by simple motivation and, thus, few treatment resources were made available. Nowadays almost all clinicians . . . agree that clinical depression needs treatment . . . Perhaps administrators, clinicians *and the public understanding of nicotine* in the 1990s is where the understanding of depression was in the early 1900s.' [8, p. 324, emphasis by the author].

Fast growth can also be seen in the drug treatment systems in most countries at the expense of treatment resources available for alcohol abusers. In Switzerland, for example, the treatment network for approximately 30 000 drug abusers, compared with the counselling and care services available to more than eight times that number of alcohol abusers, is disproportionately well developed and differentiated [9].

The images of addiction and prevailing drug, alcohol, or tobacco policies will also largely determine the type of treatment method and model. Most prominently, harm reduction measures, heroin prescription, and large-scale substitution or replacement therapies are available in all countries. Their diffusion and adoption will depend on a number of endogenous and exogenous influences such as the moral judgement of the population and adherence to international drug control [9, 10].

But even if we assume equality in the objective availability of professional help at a given time in a given country, peoples' perception of the availability of treatment still may vary and therefore affect the probability that they may look for their own solution and not seek professional assistance. In part, barriers to treatment will depend on the ability of treatment providers to tailor their services to the needs of potential clients. Natural-recovery research provides valuable information on the question as to why people do not seek treatment. Lack of information, stigma, and the belief that treatment does not offer what is needed are some of the main reasons [5, 11]. Another important reason is culturally supported beliefs. For example, Western ethics and cultural values strengthen the idea that everybody has to overcome a problem ideally without affecting others, (i.e. individual will-power and strength), downplaying the influence of other circumstances.

To conclude, the relationship between the availability of treatment resources and the prevalence of natural recovery is complex. If the treatment resources are abundant but not adapted to the needs of the clients, then the relationship will be weak or positive. A negative relationship may occur if the available treatment is plentiful and easily adapted to the needs of clients, leaving little reason to change on one's own and discouraging the use of supportive lay help. Ways to reach a balance between treatment and natural recovery by the use of either a bottom-up treatment strategy or stepped-care concept and broadening the range of available treatment options are discussed in detail in later chapters.

SELF-CHANGE IN THE GLOBAL VILLAGE: MEDIA IMAGES AND HEALTH INFORMATION MANAGEMENT AS SOCIAL CAPITAL

Self-changers under the influence: the portrayal of alcohol and drug users in the media

The ways in which social problems are presented in print, electronic media, and other public arenas can exert considerable influence on stereotypes or the willingness to provide informal support and help. The images of smoking, alcohol use, and illicit-drug use presented on television and radio, and in the print media can be understood both as a *reflection* of, and a major *influence* on, public opinion about substance use. While, in some countries, advertisements for smoking and alcohol are subject to various restrictions, it is generally claimed that only brand-specific market shares are at stake. Although a discussion of this is beyond the scope of this book, interested readers are referred to the following reference [12]. Although there are no studies showing how advertisement exposure affects recovery, it can be speculated that self-change from nicotine and alcohol problems might be more easily accomplished where cues for use are less frequent. The role of alcohol consumption in prime time TV shows, soap operas, and movies has been examined in several studies. For example, a recent study of six British soap operas showed that 86% contained visual or verbal references to alcohol beverages, with an average of one reference for every 3.5 minutes of programming. During the programs, alcohol was consumed twice as much as soft drinks [13]. An analysis of 48 German and American soap operas and crime series shown on German television also highlights the reinforcement of positive beverage-specific social stereotypes, such as the association of 'beer and friendship' [14, p. 258]. While the impact on viewers *and potential risk groups* is methodologically difficult to assess, it can be assumed that modeling approaches based on social learning theory and using melodrama are quite efficient and possibly influence people in later stages of change [15, 16].

Lemmens *et al.* [17] have presented a content analysis of the portrayal of alcohol-related issues in the print media in five national newspapers in the US from 1985 to 1991. Most articles reported alcohol issues neutrally or negatively. Furthermore, a general shift since the 1960s was noted, characterized by emphasizing public health issues, de-emphasizing clinical aspects and stressing external environmental factors more than the bio-psychological definition of alcohol-related behavior. Such media-message changes may be more conducive to self-change by not glorifying drinking and by stressing the role of environmental rather than intrapsychic factors.

As part of an evaluation of governmental drug policy in Switzerland, a national monitoring of the print media was conducted from 1993 to 2000. This analysis concerned the content and frequency of articles published on drug-related topics and showed how much topical interest fluctuates. Whereas a first peak in the reporting activities in 1994 was related to the 'showcase' of open drug scenes, the medically controlled heroin trials dominated the debate in the following years, culminating in coverage of the controversy about the public *'Youth without Drugs'* in 1997. Since then the intensity of media reports has leveled off. However, reports on hemp production and the legalization of cannabis use have been continuously released and a recent focus on doping in sports and drug-related crime can be noted [18].

Active information retrieval and media use as a tool for self-change

Individuals involved in self-change and their friends/relatives not only are passively exposed to media messages related to substance use but also, once committed to change, may seek information to gain control of their habit. Granfield and Cloud [1] define 'human capital' as part of the 'social capital' for successful self-change: 'Human capital generally refers to the knowledge, skills and other personal attributes that can be used to achieve one's desired goals . . .'

possessing knowledge and understanding that can be drawn upon to negotiate personal difficulties.

Using 'How to . . .' books

Written material can assist people in the self-change process. In most book stores there is a 'Self-Help' section. People trying to change problem behavior such as excessive eating, sex, drinking or work can turn to some type of bibliotherapy. Self-help materials may (1) be based explicitly on the principles of self-change and stages-of-change theory; (2) help to monitor and structure personal observations (e.g., drinking occasions and quantities consumed); and (3) be of a general informative nature with no stepwise or didactic program. Self-help manuals are available both for the problem drinker and for their significant others [19]. The appeal of 'how to improve your life' books [e.g. 20 on 'ways to minimize job stress and improve conflict management' as a bestseller in the USA] is probably also due to the choice they give readers, their time flexibility, and confidentiality. Self-help material has a middle position between manuals requiring minimal contact with a therapist [21, 22] and personal diaries that help to monitor personal changes, including change in substance use.

'Thursday 3 August: 8 st. 11, thigh circumference 18 inches (honestly what is bloody point), alcohol units 0, cigarettes 25 (excellent considering), negative thoughts: approx. 445 per hour, positive thoughts 0.' Bridget Jones's diary [23].

Using the Internet and cyber hugs

Personal computers are now routine items in homes and business. Worldwide it is estimated that over 113 million computers were sold in 1999 (PC World, 2000). The age group that makes the most purchases as well as being the most computer-literate (19–34 years old) also has the highest rate of risky, hazardous drinking. The Internet is a very large market for health-related information, as shown by the fact that at least 60 million people sought such information in 1998 [24]. The demand for health-related information is becoming the number one use of the Internet [25]. Further, the market for health-oriented websites is expected to increase eight-fold over five years (i.e. 1999–2004) [26]. All kinds of health information and related discussions lists [27, 28], chat rooms or cyber self-help groups on the Internet are becoming increasingly popular for many providers [29]. These sources can also be tapped by individuals trying to change their substance-use problem on their own. A big advantage for many self-quitters is the anonymity and the possibility to compare advice. Wright's [30] study on website advice for children with chronic fatigue syndrome shows that there is considerable contradictory advice on the websites. Winker *et al.* summarize the implications and problem of the Internet in this context as follows: 'Access to medical information via the Internet has the potential to speed the transformation of the patient-physician relationship from that of physician authority ministering advice and treatment to that of shared decision making between patient and physician. However, barriers impeding this transformation include wide variations in quality of content on the Web, potential for commercial interests to influence online content, and uncertain preservation of personal privacy' [31]. Young people and individuals living in remote areas are probably most inclined to use the Internet to improve their health status and possibly to handle problems with addictive behavior. As reflected in the Appendix to this book, there are numerous websites for addiction information and counselling, e.g. Smart Recovery, Web of Addiction, Moderation Management, and NHS Direct Online [32].

Lastly, as with popular self-help books, the use of the Internet is affected by social strata, age, and education [33]. The possibility to easily retrieve health-related information from the net is by no means equally distributed among either societal groups or countries: In the USA, representing 4.7% of the world population, 26.3% use the Internet. In the remaining OECD countries, with 14.7% of the world population, 6.9% are linked to the web. In Eastern Europe, which has 5.8% of the world population, Internet use is almost non-existent (0.4% users) [34]. This distribution of access to self-change-related information is in inverse proportion to the needs and the development of treatment systems in these regions.

Using research-related media calls

A relatively rare and different use of the media for self-change is to respond to advertisements. Media recruitment has been the most frequently used strategy by researchers to gain access to the hidden group of self-changers [35]. This recruitment strategy mobilizes individuals who consider themselves remitters. An often-reported reason for participation in these studies is to help others, [36]. One might speculate that talking about the recovery process to a researcher strengthens the resolution/maintenance process. Like the AA-talking cure, these accounts may serve the same purpose of confirming as well as obtaining expert confirmation of one's changed identity. A German study, comparing media and survey solicitations of self-changers, supports the idea that a research interview could serve as a way to foster maintenance. Individuals who had recovered from a more severe alcohol career responded mainly to media calls, while less severe cases were more frequently found in the survey sample. Also, the media-recruited subjects typically reported pride as a major reason for not seeking professional treatment [37].

MEDIA CAMPAIGNS SETTING THE STAGE FOR CHANGE?

Drug, alcohol and smoking campaigns are launched to sensitize the public and to influence attitudes and behavior patterns of risk groups. Similar to the question: 'How does the amount of advertising influence consumption?' is the question: 'How are the motivation for and chances of self-change affected by national sensitization campaigns?' Regrettably, Wilde's conclusion – from a decade ago – asserts that mass communication prevention programs for health are hardly ever systematically evaluated, a criticism that is still valid today [38].

Conceptual shortcomings and a lack of theoretical underpinning are seldom identified as reasons for failure. Slater has suggested that the stages-of-change model could provide a framework for integrating theories of media effects on self and others and prove to be useful for the planning of communication campaigns to change health behavior [39].

More specifically, relevant theories of the transition from pre-contemplation to contemplation are agenda setting, situational theory, and multi-step flow, which lead to interpersonal discussion of the problem behavior. Initial awareness can be built by using simple sources and dramatic messages. Moving from contemplation to preparation assumes the acceptance of the campaign messages and the perception of models and skills illustrated in engaging narrative or entertainment programming (social learning theory). Finally, the iterative process from preparation to action requires continued messages that help maintain the motivation and keep the behavior salient. Providing harder evidence, increasing language intensity, and using more directive messages have been useful for probing behavior change. At the same time this may cause resistance from self-changers who are not ready to change [39]. The stage-specific definition of campaign objectives tailoring message content accordingly and using stages of change as the primary basis of audience segmentation seems to be a promising avenue for promoting natural recovery.

However, the stages-of-change model to integrate theories that address health communication campaigns in general and facilitate self-change of problem behavior has rarely been used in the addiction field.

In this section, three Swiss campaigns, in which ideas and findings from natural-recovery research have been used as conceptual signposts, will be briefly described: (a) the 1997 drug campaign, 'A sober look at drugs', referred to *self-efficacy*; (b) the 1999 alcohol campaign, 'Handle with care', used a *stages of change* approach; and (c) the 1999/2000 tobacco campaign 'Milestone' focused on significant *life events* as agents of self-change. As part of an experimental approach to drug policies [9], the prevention debate in Switzerland has moved from a traditional substance-specific informational approach toward an orientation to health promotion and empowerment of the individual to cope successfully with life's challenges. The focus has shifted to protective factors (e.g. people's belief in having control over their lives; confidence in other people; trust in one's ability to overcome setbacks; seeing difficulties as a positive challenge; finding meaningful objectives in life). From this approach, prevention is viewed as a concern of society as a whole. From then, key elements and ideas from natural-recovery research can be used for campaigns based on this kind of thinking.

'A sober look at drugs'

The Federal Drug Sensitizing Campaigns, which started in 1991, set out to promote a better understanding of drug issues among the public at large, and included several studies: (a) a seven-year follow up of heroin users conducted by the Zurich Institute for Addiction Research [40]; (b) natural-recovery studies on alcohol and heroin remitters by the Swiss Institute for the Prevention of Alcohol and Drug Problems [5]; and (c) an epidemiological survey among heroin and cocaine users done by the University of Bern [41]. These three studies provided empirical data and were used by the campaign organizers to make their point. The national poster campaign launched in 1997 under the theme: '*A sober look at drugs*' tried to change the attitude 'once an addict always an addict', gave information about the chances of stopping drug use, and tried to strengthen hope and optimism with the slogan 'Getting into drugs does not mean to stay with them – Most drug users succeed in quitting their habit' (Figure 1).

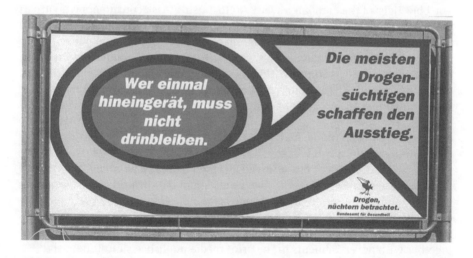

Figure 1   Campaign poster 'A sober look at drugs'

Even though annual campaign budgets of these studies (about 2 million US dollars) were low compared with commercial advertising, the objectives could be reached. A representative survey conducted in 1997 showed a positive reaction and a good recall rate, of about 31%, for that year's campaign: 52% of respondents knew someone with a drug problem. The (stigma relevant) perceived rate of drug users quitting rose from 18% in 1996 to 29% in 1997 [42]. Those directly concerned with the problem preferred the more direct and specific message: '*Coercion is no help most of the time but with our support most drug users will manage to quit*'.

This is consistent with Slater's stage-specific recommendations for media campaigns mentioned earlier. Taken together, self-efficacy and mobilizing social support for self-change were at the center of this campaign.

'Handle with care'

The alcohol campaign '*Handle with care*' is the first ever large-scale alcohol prevention program. It is sponsored by the Swiss Alcohol Board, the Swiss Office for Public Health and the Swiss Institute for the Prevention of Alcohol and Other Drug Problems (SIPA) as part of the National Alcohol Program 1998–2002. It went a step farther than the campaign 'A sober look at drugs' and adopted as theoretical underpinning a simple '*stages-of-change model*' [43] based upon the results of a representative survey ($n = 1600$) conducted in November of 1998. The objectives of the campaign were: (a) to 'push' at-risk consumers who are in the pre-contemplative phase gently forward to the contemplation stage; and (b) to influence motivated at-risk consumers to move on to the action phase.

Extrapolating the figures of this survey to the Swiss population (about 7 million) it would be estimated that not quite one million are non-drinkers, almost half are low-risk consumers (1 drink per day), about 100 000 are chronic at-risk consumers (2 or 3 drinks daily), not quite a million are episodic drinkers (bingers, 5+ or 4+ per occasion during the last month), and about 200 000 are consumers who combine heavy use and binging. The distribution across consumption patterns and stages shows that 84% of all respondents are in the pre-contemplation stage, 6.5% in the contemplation stage and a remarkable 9.5% in the action stage. Male drinkers thought about their drinking more than women, while age and linguistic region were not related to the stage progression. The 'Handle with care' logo is a bottle opener which is repeated in all messages and incorporated since July 1999 in billboard poster campaigns together with advertisements in the print media published simultaneously.

Five 18-second TV spots labeled 'minor mishaps' – situational cues – began to be shown on all Swiss TV channels and non-Swiss channels with Swiss advertising slots in March 1999. These spots featured everyday scenes showing self-confident individuals consuming alcohol and ending up with a minor mishap, or expressed differently:

A man starts to pour a glass of wine but misses the glass (*wet socks* clip), a woman burping at a ladies' tea party (*burp clip*), a man dropping ashes from a cigar into the glass of another guest (*ashes clip*), a man falling off the chair (*falling clip*), and a woman almost going to the men's toilet (*wrong door clip*). All situations are in non-dramatic and leisure time settings. The spot ends with the question on the screen '*Everything under control?*' prompting viewers to question if their alcohol consumption is maybe a bit problematic and should be given more thought [44, 45].

An evaluation based on a representative population survey ($n = 1258$) conducted in August/September 1999 showed that the acceptance (90%) and credibility (78%) of the campaign were very high. Twenty-two percent of the respondents reported that the campaign made them think about their own alcohol consumption, and 38% believed that 'Handle with care' would generate general concern about alcohol [46]. According to the report the impact on the male population and subjects in the action phase was stronger than for female respondents and pre-contemplators. The impact varied also as a function of the different types of communication (e.g. TV-spots, billboards). About a third of the interviewees spoke about the campaign and its topic with others [46] which, according to Slater, is likely to influence perceived social norms and expectations concerning the behavior, as well as impact salience directly [39]. How much success these results indicate could only be determined in comparison with other campaigns and taking other elements of the campaign into consideration: '*Handle with Care*' targets the population segment progressing to the action stage-promoting also self-monitoring material in tune with the principles of 'assisted self-change' and 'minimal intervention'. To monitor one's own alcohol consumption a handy '*alcohol slide-ruler*' is given away in physicians' waiting rooms and at counseling agencies (Figure 2).

An interview guideline for early detection is distributed among physicians and the development of drinking diaries, a handbook on early detection in primary care, and specific training courses is under way [47]. However, even in such a large-scale campaign the successful matching of content and stage-specific target groups still needs to be systematically evaluated.

'Few campaigns are large or comprehensive enough to attempt to address each stage (of change) systematically in a single coordinated effort. Most focus on key populations at two or three stage points. When resources are limited, as in most campaigns, this may be a good idea. This need to focus is particularly true, I think, in substance-abuse-oriented efforts. Prevention versus treatment and addressing potential users versus actual users represent quite disparate tasks.' [48].

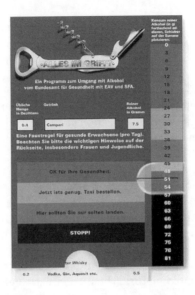

Figure 2   Tools for assisted self-change: 'The alcohol slide ruler'

Milestone

'A lifestyle is born – MILESTONE the most pleasurable non-smoking campaign since we know cigarettes' was launched in 1999 by the Swiss Cancer League and the Swiss Office of Public Health. The concept of the 'milestone' is based on *significant life* events that trigger spontaneous remission, a classic theme of natural recovery (Figure 3). Key elements are 'the special moments which make life worthwhile and break through the daily routine: the first child, the pompous wedding, the new sports car, the trip around the world, the dream job, the successful exam, the important birthday, the new apartment with view on the lake ...'. MILESTONE symbolizes the end of a phase in your life and a new beginning ...' (Press release, 21 October 1999, Bern, Swiss Cancer League, Federal Office of Public Health).

The campaign is aiming specifically at 50% of Swiss dissonant smokers in the contemplation phase and would like 'to provide chronic smokers with the energy necessary to quit'. It is the first campaign in Switzerland that is primarily Internet-based (www.yourmilestone.ch); it also uses a telephone hotline and information material.

This is how it works. First, smokers sign up on the website and define their *'personal milestone'*, which is a date and an event marking the start of the attempt to quit smoking. This is part of a public data base *'portraits'* with all the participants. Second, they receive an e-mail on the date reminding them of their intention. Third, after three months participants receive another e-mail to

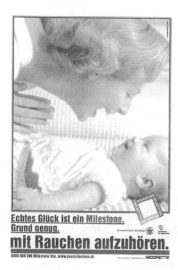 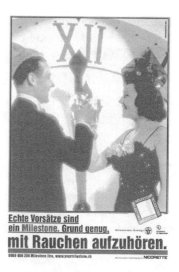

Figure 3   Life events as 'personal milestones' to quit smoking

report 'failure or success'. Fourth, reported successes are filed under 'congratulations' and 'the winners' receive a gift. Reported 'failures' are encouraged to resubscribe by choosing another milestone. During the phase of remission, the website offers tools for 'assisted self-change' such as information on nicotine replacement, self-help groups and self-monitoring devices. The principle of social modeling is introduced by the presentation of VIPs under the category *'your idols'* who are supporting the campaign and trying themselves to quit. Social support is mobilized in two ways: (1) with *'your friends'* an electronic e-mail postcard can be forwarded to a smoker by a friend offering a direct link to the web site, and (2) 'your opinion' offers a chat room for people commenting on the smoking in general or encouraging specific individuals in the portrait data base.

The success of the Milestone campaign will be evaluated by telephone surveys and personal interviews in groups as well with a quantitative and qualitative analysis of the website visits. After about 100 days, 300 people had signed up with a personal milestone. During the first three months the website had 25 000 visitors who stayed an average of four minutes; 18 000 down-loaded the non-smoking questionnaire [49, 50]. The network approach of the campaign also builds on the personnel managers of partner companies who actively promote the Olympic game *'Fit for Sydney'* at the workplace beginning on 19 April 2000. Small teams of two would-be quitters and *two non-smokers as coaches* have the opportunity to collect miles per days without smoking and to qualify for a lottery to win a trip to Sydney. The positive 'trendy' brandmark of this campaign is only geared to positive life events and personal landmarks. It will be interesting to analyse the negative and critical 'personal milestones' that are mentioned in the Internet admission forms and compare this information with natural-recovery research and stage-specific findings.

STRUCTURAL PREVENTION AND CHANCES OF CHANGE: 'HOW FAR IS IT TO THE NEXT PUB?'

Availability of alcohol and drugs is subject to change and may vary greatly between societies, groups, and regions. Taxation policies and various degrees of competition on drug markets will influence prices and consumption patterns, [51, 52]. Most of the discussion in the natural-recovery field has focused on general consumption levels rather than on the effects of the addiction problem on individual behavior. How sensitive are drug abusers in different stages of change to price change? Are substitution processes (i.e. one drug for another) affected by differential prices, health policies or income fluctuations? In this context Godfrey points out interesting implications of Becker and Murphy's [53] economic model of rational addiction for self-change processes:

> '... permanent changes in prices may have small short-run effects, but the long run demand for addictive goods is predicted to be more elastic than the demand for non-addictive goods. Some addictive behavior patterns such as 'binges', *abrupt discontinuity of consumption, and repeated quitting behavior* (emphasis by the author) are also consistent with this model of 'rational' behavior' [54, p. 180].

Self-reward schemes of quitters (spending the money I saved for something else I like) and the pressure to quit because of the increasing financial burden to keep up the habit could serve as examples of how these environmental conditions can affect individual behavior (see also Chapter 9 on price changes).

Contextual conditions for change are by no means stable over time and across countries. For example, conditions for self-change have been altered in the Nordic countries with the erosion of the Nordic alcohol monopolies after those countries joined the European Union [55]. In 2000 the European Commission refused to extend exemption clauses for Sweden, which limited alcohol imports.

Comparing the USA and Canada in 1989/1990, Giesbrecht and Greenfield found a greater polarization of opinion within both countries on policy items relating to promotion of alcohol or control of physical, demographic or economic access, and virtually no polarization with regard to curtailing service to drunken customers or *providing information on* treatment [56]. Within the same country, the definition of alcohol-related social harm and ideas regarding what should be done about it also can vary over time, such as the trend studies in the Netherlands. For example, Bongers, Goor and Garretsen define social climate on alcohol as '... the blend of different views on drinking, conceptions of alcohol-related problems, and the defining of appropriate measures for dealing with them ...' [57, p. 141]. The study dealt with, among other things, *tolerance towards drinking behavior of close relatives and drinking behavior at a party*, and found that tolerance increased between 1958 and 1994. Furthermore, it was found that support for advertisement restrictions and higher prices for alcoholic beverages in the Dutch population was fading [57, p. 144].

Taking another example from Switzerland, a recent liberalization of the markets has opened the way for *longer* opening hours, abolished the so-called 'need-clause' (limiting the number of outlets as a function of the population) and led to the introduction of unified tax rates for distilled spirits after a ruling of the World Trade Organisation in July 1999. The British Government also plans to reform the licensing regulations even though national opinion polls do not necessarily show public support for such a policy [58–60]. Ironically, recent American studies have highlighted the potential merits of structural alcohol prevention and restrictions in the community. Scribner's study in 24 urban residential tracts in New Orleans investigated the effect the number of retail alcohol outlets (liquor, grocery and convenience stores) had on individual attitudes towards drinking and alcohol consumption. They found that certain neighborhoods had an over-concentration of alcohol outlets (i.e. 5 per 3000 people). Not surprisingly, alcohol consumption in these areas was 11% higher. Although it is impossible to know whether the number of outlets increased regional consumption or were responding to pre-existing regional demands, especially interesting with respect to self-change is the correlation of these environmental conditions with attitudes of family members. Views toward drinking were 15% to 16% more favorable than in residential tracts with lower outlet density [61].

'This result is very different from what we had believed, that everyone's individual behavior was controlled by just their individual character-istics. But now we see that the neighborhood that people live in counts for a significant portion of their individual behavior. That's huge. In the last four or five years, people in community organizations in cities such as Los Angeles, Washington, New Orleans, Oakland and Chicago have become aware of a link between higher densities of alcohol outlets and higher incidences of alcohol-related outcomes' (Dr. Richard Scribner, Professor of Prevention Medicine, Louisiana State University – Health Services Center; interview with *Medical Tribune* 15 February 2000).

To conclude, individuals pursuing self-change are members of local drinking cultures. Because 'alcohol outlets in a neighborhood are dynamically linked to the social network in which interdependent actors carry out their daily activities' [62, p. 310], these conditions can represent major stumbling blocks on the way to recovery.

DISCUSSION: MOTIVATION TO CHANGE AND REFERENCES TO SOCIETY

Most of the contextual references (i.e. environmental features) discussed in this chapter often do not show up in the narrative accounts presented in natural-recovery research. Most likely, individuals when interviewed about why 'they' recovered will not make reference to 'society', 'outlet density' or similar macro-concepts. This could be an artefact and a consequence of the individualistic bias described in the introduction. However, this does not mean that the macro-societal factors outlined in this chapter do not have an effect on the change process at the individual level. Identity transformation processes do become visible when people talk about religious and spiritual experiences as the causes of their recovery and when they assume professional roles as helpers to foster their change and make good use of their deviant expertise in the past for respectable roles [63]. Multiple identity theory, assuming that 'with each social world (or social group) membership comes an identity and each identity has a particular perspective or viewpoint on the world as well as prescriptions for thought and behavior' [64. p. 235] could therefore be a promising perspective for a better understanding of societal factors in the natural recovery process.

REFERENCES

1. Granfield, R. and Cloud, W. (1999) *Coming Clean: Overcoming Addiction Without Treatment*, New York University Press: New York.
2. Oldenburg, B., Glanz, K. and French, M. (1999) The application of staging models to the understanding of health behavior change and the promotion of health. *Psychol Health* 14, 503–516.
3. Müller, R. and Weiss, W. (1984) *Das Bild des Alkoholikers in der Öffentlichkeit*, Schweizerische Fachstelle für Alkoholprobleme: Lausanne.
4. Fahrenkrug, H. (1992) Alkohol: Laster oder Krankheit. *Schweizer Apothekerzeitung* 20(8), 593–595.
5. Klingemann, H.K.H. (1992) Coping and maintenance strategies of spontaneous remitters from problem use of alcohol and heroin in Switzerland. *Int J Addict.* 27, 1359–1388.
6. Cunningham, J.A., Sobell, L.C. and Sobell, M.B. (1998) Awareness of self-change as a pathway to recovery for alcohol abusers: Results from five different groups. *Addict Behav.* 23(3), 399–404.
7. Kavanagh, D.J., Sitharthan, T., Spilsbury, G. and Vignaedra, S. (1999) An evaluation of brief correspondence programs for problem drinkers. *Behav Ther.* 30, 641–656.

8. Hughes, J.R. (1999) Four beliefs that may impede progress in the treatment of smoking. *Tob Control* **8**, 323–326.
9. Klingemann, H. and Hunt, G. (1998) *Drug Treatment Systems in An International Perspective*, Sage Publications Inc.: Thousand Oaks, CA.
10. Klingemann, H. and Klingemann, H.-D. (1999) National treatment systems in global perspective. *Eur Addict Res.* **5**, 109–117.
11. Klingemann, H.K.-H. (1991) The motivation for change from problem alcohol and heroin use. *Br J Addict.* **86**, 727–744.
12. Godfrey, C. (1986) Government policy, advertising and tobacco consumption in the UK: A critical review of the literature. *Br J Addict.* **81**, 339–346.
13. Furnham, A., Hingle, H. and Gunter, B.A.M. (1997) A content analysis of alcohol portrayal and drinking in British television soap operas. *Health Educ Res.* **12**(4), 519–529.
14. Weiderer, M. (1997) Aspects of alcohol drinking and alcohol abuse in soap-operas and crime series of German Television. *Sucht* **43**(4), 254–263.
15. Slater, M.D. (1997) Persuasion processes across receiver goals and message genres. *Commun Theory* **7**, 125–148.
16. Rogers, E.M., Vaughan, P. and Shefner-Rogers, C.L. (1995) Evaluating the effects of an entertainment-education radio soap opera in Tanzania: A field experiment with multi-method measurement, in *Annual Conference of the International Communication Association, May 1995*, Albuquerque, New Mexico, 1995.
17. Lemmens, P.H., Vaeth, P.A.C. and Greenfield, T.K. (1999) Coverage of beverage alcohol issues in the print media in the United States, 1985–1991. *Am J Public Health* **89**(10), 1555–1560.
18. Boller, B. (1999) Übersicht Drogenberichterstattung der Schweizer Presse. Institut für Journalistik und Kommunikationswissenschaft, Universität Fribourg, Fribourg.
19. Barber, J.G. and Gilbertson, R. (1998) Evaluation of a self-help manual for the female partners of heavy drinkers. *Res Social Work Pract.* **8**(2), 141–151.
20. Carlson, R. (1998) *Don't Sweat the Small Stuff at Work*, Hyperion: New York.
21. Heather, N. (1986) *Change Without Therapists: The Use of Self-help Manual by Problem Drinkers*, Pergamon: New York.
22. Noschis, K. (1988/89) Testing a self-help instrument with early-risk alcohol consumers in general practice: A progress report. *Contemp Drug Probl.* **15**, 365–381.
23. Fielding, H. (1996) *Bridget Jones's Diary*, Picador – MacMillan: London.
24. Kaufman, M. (1999) The Internet: A reliable source? Washington Post, February 16, Section Z17.
25. Intel. (2000) Online survey shows details of health content retrievers, in <www.intel.com./intel/e-health/jdpower.htm>, January 7, 2000.
26. Intellihealth. (2000) Online health spending to soar, in <http://ipn.intelihealth.com/ipn/ihtIPN?st=719&c=264078>, January 30, 2000.
27. McCartney, P.R. (1999) Internet communication and discussion lists for perinatal nurses. *J Perinat Neonatal Nurs.* **12**(4), 26–40.
28. Moran, M.L. (1999) Dissemination of geriatric rehabilitation information via the Internet. *Top Geriatr Rehabil.* **14**(3), 80–85.
29. Wiley, D.L. (1999) Health information on the Internet by B. Maxwell. *Online* **23**(2), 94–95.
30. Wright, B., Williams, C. and Partridge, I. (1999) Management advice for children with chronic fatigue syndrome: a systematic study of information from the internet. *Irish J Psychol Med.* **16**(2), 67–71.

31. Winker, M.A., Flanagin, A., Chi-Lum, B. *et al.* (2000) Guidelines for medical and health information sites on the Internet – Principles governing AMA web sites. *JAMA.* **283**, 1600–1606.
32. Alcohol Alert. (2000) Advice on-line. *Alcohol Alert* (1), 8–9.
33. Korgaonkar, P.K. and Wolin, L.D. (1999) A multivariate analysis of Web usage. *Journal of Advertising Research* **39**(2), 53–68.
34. Uimonen, P. (2000) Gegen Zensur und Unterdrückung im Internet. *Deutschland Zeitschrift für Politik, Kultur, Wirtschaft und Wissenschaft*, 62–65.
35. Sobell, L.C., Ellingstad, T.P. and Sobell, M.B. (2000) Natural recovery from alcohol and drug problems: Methodological review of the research with suggestions for future directions. *Addiction* **95**, 749–769.
36. Sobell, L.C., Sobell, M.B. and Toneatto, T. (1992) Recovery from alcohol problems without treatment, in *Self-Control and the Addictive Behaviours* (eds. N. Heather, W.R. Miller and J. Greeley), Maxwell MacMillan: New York, pp. 198–242.
37. Rumpf, H.-J., Bischof, G., Hapke, U., Meyer, C. and John, U. (2000) Studies on natural recovery from alcohol dependence: Sample selection bias by media solicitation. *Addiction* **95**, 747.
38. Wilde, G.J.S. (1991) Effects of mass media communications upon health and safety habits of individuals: an overview of issues and evidence. *Addictions* **88**, 983–996.
39. Slater, M.D. (1999) Integrating application of media effects, persuasion and behavior change theories to communication campaigns: a stages-of-change framework. *Health Commun.* **11**, 335–354.
40. Dobler-Mikola, A., Zimmer Höfler, D., Uchtenhagen, A. and Korbel, R. (1991) Soziale Integration und Desintegration in der 7-Jahreskatamnese bei (ehemals) Heroinabhängigen. Forschungsinformation aus dem Sozialpsychiatrischen Dienst: Zurich, Report no. 38.
41. Estermann, J., Herrmann, U., Hügi, D. and Nydegger, B. (1996) Zusammenfassung der wichtigsten Ergebnisse-Empfehlungen, in *Sozialepidemiologie des Drogenkonsums* (ed. J. Estermann), Verlag für Wissenschaft und Bildung: Berlin, pp. 155–162.
42. Moeri, R. (1997) Auswertung der Kurzevaluation zur Kampagne 'Drogen, nüchtern betrachtet – Eine Mehrheit beurteilt die Kampagne positiv. *BAG Bulletin* 42.
43. Prochaska, J.O. and DiClemente, C.C. (1986) Toward a comprehensive model of change, in Treating Addictive Behaviors: Processes of Change (eds. W.E. Miller and N. Heather), Plenum: New York, pp. 3–27.
44. Spectra. (1999) Petits malheurs. *Spectra* **15**, 8.
45. Spectra. (1999) Un million de personnes ont un comportement risqué avec l'alcool. *Spectra* **16**, 7.
46. Ronco, C. (1999) Globalevaluation Alcoholprogramm 1999–2002: Posttest der Kampagne 'Alles im Griff?', Dübendorf: IPSO September 1999.
47. Stahl, S. and Brenner, D.E. (1999) 'Alles im Griff?' zählt auf die Aertzteschaft. *Newsletter SGA* **4**, 17–18.
48. Slater, M. (2000) Personal communication, Colorado State University, March 10, 2000.
49. Schweizerische Krebsliga. (2000) Fact sheet – Evaluation 100 Tage Milestone, in Schweizerische Krebsliga: Bern.
50. Siegenthaler, U. (2000) Jedem Projekt seine eigene Website? Der Erfolg der Milestone – Website weckt neue Gelüste. *Krebsliga intern* (1), 11–12.
51. Österberg, E. (1992) Effects of alcohol control measures on alcohol consumption. *Int J Addict.* **27**, 209–225.
52. Klingemann, H.K.H. (1994) Environmental influences which promote or impede change in substance behaviour, in *Addiction: Processes of Change* (eds G. Edwards and M. Lader), Oxford University Press: Oxford, pp. 131–161.

53. Becker, G.S. and Murphy, K.M. (1988) A theory of rational addiction. *J Political Econ.* **96**, 675–700.
54. Godfrey, C. (1994) Economic influences on change in population and personal substance behaviour, in *Addiction: Processes of Change* (eds G. Edwards and M. Lader), Oxford University Press: Oxford, pp. 163–187.
55. Holder, H., Kühlhorn, E., Nordlund, S., Oesterberg, E., Romelsjö, A. and Trygve, U. *European Integration and Nordic Alcohol Policies – Changes in Alcohol Controls and Consequences in Finland, Norway and Sweden 1980–1997*, Ashgate: Aldershot.
56. Giesbrecht, N. and Greenfield, T.K. (1999) Public opinion on alcohol policy issues: A comparison of American and Canadian surveys. *Addiction* **94**(4), 521–531.
57. Bongers, I.M.B., Goor, I.A.M. and Garretsen, H.F.L. (1998) Social climate on alcohol in Rotterdam, the Netherlands: Public opinion on drinking behaviour and alcohol measures. *Alcohol Alcohol* **32**(2), 141–150.
58. Alcohol Alert. (2000) Alcohol policy – what the public thinks. *Alcohol Alert* (1), 2–4.
59. Alcohol Alert. (2000) Minister lays down the law. *Alcohol Alert* (1), 6.
60. Alcohol Alert. (2000) White Paper. *Alcohol Alert* (1), 7.
61. Scribner, R.A., Cohen, D.A. and Fisher, W. (2000) Evidence of a structural effect for alcohol outlet density: A multi-level analysis. *Alcohol: Clin Exp Res.* **245**, 188–195.
62. Scribner, R., Cohen, D., Kaplan, S. and Allen, S.H. (1999) Alcohol availability and homicide in New Orleans: Conceptual considerations for small area analysis of the effect of alcohol outlet density. *J Stud Alcohol* **60**, 310–316.
63. Klingemann, H.K.H. (1999) Addiction careers and careers in addiction. *Subst Use Misuse* **34**(11), 1505–1526.
64. Kellog, S. (1993) Identity and recovery. *Psychotherapy* **30**, 235–243.

Chapter six

One way to leave your lover: the role of treatment in changing addictive behavior

The problem is all inside your head she said to me.
The answer is easy if you take it logically . . .
There must be fifty ways to leave your lover.
                    Paul Simon, '50 Ways to Leave Your Lover', 1975

Whether the topic is addictive behavior, infections or fractures, the traditional view of treatment in a medical model is that it addresses the cause of the disorder and either returns the person to normal functioning or helps the individual achieve a reasonable accommodation to a disability. For treatment of withdrawal symptoms, the medical model is defensible – the disorder has a known physiological basis, the treatment derives from that knowledge, and the treatment is reliably effective. For other aspects of addictive behavior, especially compulsive use, the model's fit is very questionable. The basis for the behavior is neither understood nor necessarily physiological (although drug effects have a physiological basis, this does not mean that the 'cause' of their use is physiological).

MEANINGFUL EXPLANATIONS OF CHANGE IN ADDICTIVE BEHAVIOR

Tucker and King [1] have pointed out that the effects of interventions for addictive behaviors typically are associated with short-term benefit but plagued by problem recurrence. This occurs despite the interventions being based on divergent assumptions (e.g. learned behavior, disease) and having different procedures (e.g. lengths). Outcomes are also positively associated with an individual's resources and with environmental variables following treatment. When people recover from substance abuse problems without intervention [2] such natural recoveries often are not reactions to specific precipitating events but rather follow cognitive reappraisals (also reviewed in [2], i.e. the individual weighs the pros and cons and makes a decision to change [3]). This suggests that the critical ingredient for precipitating change is an individual's commitment (i.e. motivation) to change. The viewpoint adopted in this chapter is that any meaningful explanation of change in addictive behavior (i.e. recovery) must be able to explain all varieties of change, including those stimulated by environmental events, those that have been described as the result of a 'maturing out' process, and other natural recoveries.

FIFTY WAYS TO LEAVE YOUR LOVER

Recovered Alcohol Abuser

'I wasn't a human being as I intended to be. I had reached a point where I felt trapped by alcohol. It was my mistress . . .'

An individual's attraction to a drug of choice can be understood as a love relationship [4, 5]. Taking the analogy one step further, there are many ways in which the dissolution of relationships can be achieved, many ways to leave one's lover. That there are multiple routes to recovery from substance abuse problems becomes easier to understand when the full range of problems is considered rather than an isolated focus on severe cases [6]. This issue has been best addressed for alcohol problems where epidemiological findings have indicated that the population of individuals with severe problems is far outnumbered by those with less severe problems. The Institute of Medicine in its 1990 report to the National Institute on Alcohol Abuse and Alcoholism estimated the ratio to be four not severely dependent alcohol abusers for every severely dependent case [6]. Most people do not find it surprising that persons with minor alcohol problems often overcome their problems without the assistance of others. Likewise, it is common knowledge that most people who stop smoking do so on their own [7, 8]. Also, like treated alcohol abusers, ex-smokers in treatment are more dependent than the average smoker and, before stopping smoking, ex-smokers were less dependent on nicotine than are current smokers [9]. Time and again the conclusion that makes the most sense is that change can be achieved by many routes and that the most important precipitant of change is the decision to change. In short, someone who is strongly motivated to change will find a way to do so.

Recovered Alcohol Abusers

Example 1:
'Well, basically you have to want to stop. You have to recognize that you have a problem, then you have to really want to stop. I guess there's a thing I refer to as self-esteem and if you don't have that then I think you're lost. It's going to be a barrier so you must feel that you're a good person and you can do it.

Example 2:
'Well I think I had the feeling that if I'm gonna beat this thing it's up to me, and nobody else is going to make me stop drinking. It's my problem and I have to resolve it myself. Why should I go to, and ask, somebody else and put my problems on their shoulders, when it's one of my own.?'

Example 3:
'I was supposed to take her to a Sunday School picnic in the afternoon, on that Saturday afternoon, and on that Saturday morning I got juiced up and I was unable to take her. So the next day I had a terrible feeling of guilt and remorse and I guess maybe I had one or two beers left, I gulped that, and I said this is it. That's the end of that nonsense and I've never had a drink since. Well it just happened that this was the last straw, I guess. I made up my mind that I'm going to beat this thing and this is the end of it. Good-bye! I was going to beat it. I felt so badly about it.'

Tucker [10] has compellingly argued for viewing recovery within an individual's total life context as it evolves over time. From this viewpoint, behavior change is not necessarily seen as an isolated event; it can also be the endpoint of a process that takes place over time. The onset and offset of substance abuse problems can be viewed as phases in the individual's career. The remainder of this chapter will consider why some individuals utilize treatment services as part of their attempts to change, while others do not?

Figure 1 presents a hypothetical overview of the behavior change process. Although this figure will be discussed with regard to addictive behavior, the same model could be used to describe different types of behavior change. The early part of the change process (i.e. becoming committed to change) has recently become a topic of considerable research in the addiction field. Research on motivation was fueled by Prochaska and DiClemente's [11, 12] extension of Prochaska's transtheoretical model of change in psychotherapy to the addictions field. The model breaks the change process down into a set of hypothetical stages. While the model has been the subject of considerable criticism and

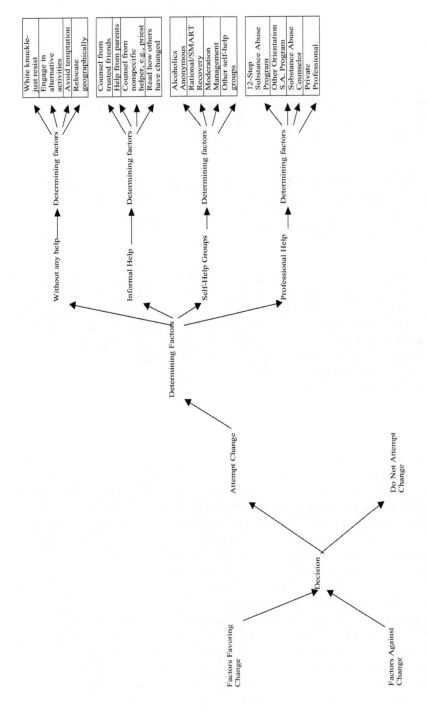

Figure 1 Overview of the behavior change process

controversy recently [13–17], a review of these issues is beyond the scope of this chapter. The important features of the model for the present consideration are (a) that it postulates that motivation is a state variable (i.e. changeable) and as such should be addressed in treatment, and (b) that it makes no sense to conduct therapy intended to help an individual change if the individual is not committed to changing.

Whereas the stages-of-change (transtheoretical) model evoked a plethora of research and comment, including the advent of motivational interviewing as an alternative approach to dealing with individuals in substance abuse treatment [18, 19], research on how change is effected, the help-seeking process, and the role of treatment in change has been neither plentiful nor well organized. This hypothetical process as presented in Figure 1 can be viewed as involving two phases: (1) deciding upon the general route of change to be followed, and (2) deciding the specific route of change. Although research and common sense make clear that alternative routes to recovery exist and are used, research is seriously deficient concerning the sets of variables labeled as 'Determining Factors' in Figure 1. Figure 1 considers the change process from the standpoint of the individual and not from the perspective of the treatment professional. Thus, the necessary research does not consist of matching research aimed at identifying what types of individual will do best in what types of treatment [20], but rather research about how people decide how they will attempt to change, whether they will seek help, what type of help they will seek, and why.

Because the focus of this chapter is on the role of treatment in change, the existing literature on factors affecting help-seeking will not be reviewed here. Moreover, reviews of that literature are already available [21–24]. Instead, this discussion will be largely conceptual, with an emphasis on identifying areas of research likely to illuminate influences on change decisions.

FACTORS INFLUENCING ROUTE OF CHANGE

Although there has been a dearth of research on how people choose their route of attempted recovery, this does not mean that the boxes labeled 'determining factors' in Figure 1 are black boxes. Some relevant research has been reported, and there are several factors that logically belong among the boxes' content. Table 1 presents a conceptual listing of factors likely to influence an individual's decision about what recovery route to pursue. These factors, which operate in selecting the general route of change and the specific method within that route, range from personal beliefs and experiences to practical issues, and to community structure and attitudes.

Having made a decision to attempt to change, the ways in which an individual can approach that objective must start from the individual's knowledge about how to change and what assistance might be available. It should be noted that this knowledge derives not only from general information and help that is

Table 1   Factors likely to influence decisions about what route of change to pursue

Information/knowledge
   Treatment programs
   How others have changed
   Self-help-group existence and local availability
   Trusted others available to provide informal counsel
   Professional services available
   How people recover from substance abuse

Environmental factors
   Availability of self-help groups, treatment programs, professionals
   Access to services (e.g. waiting lists, transportation)
   Community attitudes toward problems, recovery, etc.

Personal situation/pragmatic factors
   Cost of treatment programs, professional services
   Interference with other responsibilities (e.g. work, child care)

Psychological factors
   Attitude toward independence
   Trust of others to give aid
   Beliefs about how one should recover
   Past experiences

available but also vicariously from knowing about the experiences of others. In terms of community health service planning, it is obvious that using services efficiently will begin with the population being aware of cost-effective services and, importantly, being aware that many persons are able to recover without using formal services. Because traditional substance abuse programs tend to be intensive and costly [6, 25], at least in the US, it would be highly advisable to embark on a campaign to make the general population aware of multiple routes to recovery. Finally, there are two ways by which information plays a role in determining the route of recovery. First, it serves to constrain alternatives. People cannot be expected to adopt alternatives that they do not know exist. A second and even more important issue is that. besides knowing that alternatives are available, individuals should also have accurate information in order to make decisions among those alternatives. For example, in North America it is commonly believed that Alcoholics Anonymous and 12-Step programs have been demonstrated to be the most effective approaches to recovery, although this is at odds with the empirical literature [26]. Thus, an additional prerequisite for achieving efficient use of community services is the dissemination of accurate information about all available routes of recovery.

Environmental factors also influence decisions about which recovery routes to select. Starting with differences such as urban and rural environments, the setting will place real limits upon the substance abusers' options [27]. Environmental considerations can be greatly affected by the availability of treatment programs as well as helping professionals, since even small communities tend to have self-help groups available. However, even in very small communities, if privacy is important, then this may serve as a barrier to using self-help groups.

Recovered Alcohol Abuser

'He said, 'You're known as a town drunk.' Now there were other things that had happened as well ... But that was the cruncher. I really blew my lid when he said that. When he said that I was known as a town drunk, no son of mine or family has to put up with that from me.'

Another important aspect of the environment that impacts choosing a route of change relates to access to services [28, 29]. Factors such as convenience or difficulty in accessing services or length of time until services are available (e.g. waiting lists) may not be tolerable and may ultimately affect a person's decision to change. Also, the environment acts as a source of collective social influence [29, 30]. The individual's social network provides not only support and advice but also a context of beliefs, attitudes and hearsay about methods of change. To the extent that social approval is important to the individual, social context is bound to influence decisions about change routes.

Recovered Alcohol Abuser

'You know, one of the greatest things that happened was that (name deleted) never drank very much, but she quit and supported me ... So she decided then that 'hey, you know, I am not going to drink either.' And from that moment neither of us drank anything. Yes, cause it's a social thing.'

Individualized factors will also impact choice of alternatives. Many of the change routes extract personal costs that the individual may or may not find worthwhile. These range from monetary costs for treatment programs or professional services, to the investment of time (e.g. inpatient treatment to attending weekly self-help group meetings), to competing with responsibilities (e.g. at home or work) and activities (e.g. hobbies, gardening).

Lastly, central to choosing change routes will be psychological factors. The other factors discussed so far serve to make the individual aware of a menu of choices and a set of costs and benefits related to each choice. However, the resultant choice is made against the backdrop of psychological factors. Individual differences in traits, attitudes, backgrounds, preferences, values and the other factors that combine to yield our idiosyncratic identities will ultimately serve as the filtering mechanisms through which choice emerges. Some of these factors may include the stigma that often surrounds issues of substance abuse as well as a general fear of, or unwillingness to engage in, treatment. The latter factor also affects help-seeking for many health problems that are not stigmatizing, such as heart disease [29]. Such factors have long been ignored despite their obvious importance to understanding how people decide what methods to use in attempting to change. Understanding how people decide what route to try to change is extremely important for health care planning. It is clear that if all individuals with substance abuse problems were to seek to use treatment services the amount of services available would be woefully inadequate. Thus, while this area of research begins with observational and descriptive research, ultimately the goals would be (a) to encourage those individuals who can achieve self-change or recovery through self-help programs to do so; and (b) to promote a set of empirically-based interventions by which substance abusers can identify the services likely to be necessary to resolve their problem.

THE ROLE OF TREATMENT IN CHANGING ADDICTIVE BEHAVIOR

This section focuses on the role of treatment in changing addictive behavior and assumes that other community-level interventions are necessary to achieve the dual goals of (a) increasing the use of treatment where necessary, and (b) decreasing unnecessary use of treatment. Given the above context for help seeking, what should be the role of treatment in changing addictive behavior? One aspect of the role is to just 'be there.' For treatment to be a route to change, opportunities for treatment must exist. In an ideal world, it would be sufficient to make a variety of services available which could be utilized according to need. However, need for assistance in changing may be only one reason why people utilize clinical services. For example, Breslin [personal communication, November 1999], found that several participants who had successful outcomes in a brief intervention trial nevertheless went on to use additional services in the community. This may have been because, although their outcomes were positive from a research perspective (i.e. in terms of substance use), they continued to have associated problems (e.g. interpersonal), because they felt they needed help maintaining the changes they had accomplished, or because of other reasons. Aasland *et al.* [31] have suggested that some people enter addiction treatment after they have already changed, with the purpose of treatment being to maintain the change. Whatever the reason, perceptions of the need for treatment may differ markedly from the views of professionals. If such services are paid for by the individuals themselves, this is less of a problem than services that are reimbursed by public programs or insurance providers. Thus, besides having a variety of services available, there also is a need to provide triage services to assure that funds are spent wisely to provide necessary care.

STEPPED-CARE APPROACH

One way of providing services efficiently would be for the substance abuse field to embrace a stepped-care model of service provision [32]. Such an approach is shown in Figure 2 and reflects how services are delivered for many health problems. It requires providers to abide by certain guidelines in making treatment recommendations, with the initial recommendations based both on empirically-based knowledge and on clinical judgment. The guidelines are that the treatment of choice should be (1) individualized, (2) consistent with the contemporary research literature, (3) least restrictive but still likely to work, and (4) acceptable to the consumer. Following the initial treatment disposition, decisions about further treatment are performance-based, i.e. they depend upon whether the individual shows a good response to treatment. If the response to treatment is inadequate, consideration is given to stepping up the care to be more intensive or to using a different approach. For example, in the treatment of hypertension, typically a family physician is likely to recommend various lifestyle changes such as exercise and diet as first treatment of choice, followed by medication, and eventual referral to a specialist if the previous interventions are not effective. Accumulating evidence suggests that individuals who will do well with brief cognitive-behavioral treatment will show substantial change within the first few sessions of treatment [33]. Thus, individuals who do not show early change might be good candidates for stepping up the level of services.

MULTIPLE FUNCTIONS OF TREATMENT

Finally, in terms of the functions that can be served by treatment, several general themes are evident. Treatment can serve as an opportunity for people to organize their thoughts about their problems and make informed decisions about priorities. This may be one reason why motivational enhancement treatments incorporate decisional balancing exercises compelling the individual to weigh the pros and cons of changing or of staying the same [19]. Another function of treatment can be to help people understand their predicament and how they got there and to give hope that change is possible. In some cases, when people become aware of the relationship between precipitating factors and

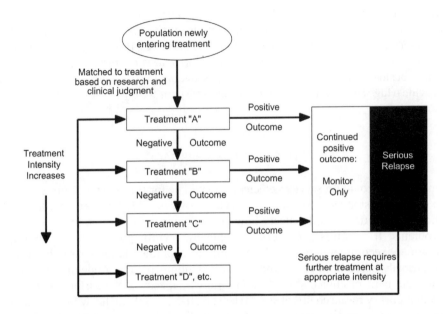

Figure 2 Stepped care model of health service delivery. Adapted from [34] with permission of the authors

consequences and their substance use, this may be sufficient for them to initiate change, while in other cases change may be difficult, or impossible, without the acquisition of necessary skills. Another potential function of treatment is to provide social support and reinforcement for change, especially if clients lack such resources as part of their everyday environment. Lastly, treatment can 'buy time' for people. For example, individuals who are under social pressure to change, but not yet ready to change, could enter treatment and attend sessions to satisfy others, but have no intention of changing their substance use.

SUMMARY: MANY WAYS TO LEAVE YOUR LOVER

It is evident that change in substance use can be accomplished in many ways, with treatment being only one way. This chapter was intended to provide an organizational framework for conceptualizing variables important for precipitating change. Although the multiple components of change were described conceptually rather than reviewed, an important point that this chapter highlighted is that little is known about factors determining (1) how a person decides to try to change, (2) why and when someone seeks help, and (3) how one chooses among alternatives, including treatment. Research on client-treatment matching will be of limited benefit without corresponding research on (a) getting clients to select treatments that are likely to be least restrictive but nevertheless effective, as well as (b) research on getting service providers to adopt a professional, stepped-care approach to service provision rather than being wed to services developed for severe cases (and therefore too intensive for individuals with less severe problems) [6, 10].

REFERENCES

1. Tucker, J.A. and King, M.P. (1999) Resolving alcohol and drug-related problems: Influences on behavior change and help-seeking processes, in *Changing Addictive Behavior: Bridging Clinical and Public Health Strategies* (eds J.A. Tucker, D.A. Donovan and G.A. Marlatt), Guilford Press: New York, pp. 97–126.
2. Sobell, L.C., Ellingstad, T.P. and Sobell, M.B. (2000) Natural recovery from alcohol and drug problems: Methodological review of the research with suggestions for future directions. *Addiction* 95, 749–769.
3. Sobell, L.C., Sobell, M.B., Toneatto, T. and Leo, G.I. (1993) What triggers the resolution of alcohol problems without treatment? *Alcohol: Clin Exp Res.* 17(2), 217–224.
4. Saunders, B. and Allsop, S. (1985) Giving up addictions, in *New Developments in Clinical Psychology* (ed. F.N. Watts), John Wiley: New York, pp. 203–220.
5. Stewart, T. (1987) *The Heroin Users*, Pandora Press: London.
6. Institute of Medicine. (1990) *Broadening the Base of Treatment for Alcohol Problems*, National Academy Press: Washington, D.C.
7. Fiore, M.C., Novotny, T.E., Pierce, J.P. *et al.* (1990) Methods used to quit smoking in the United States. *JAMA.* 263, 2760–2765.
8. Orleans, C.T., Schoenbach, V.J., Wagner, E.H., *et al.* (1991) Self-help quit smoking interventions: Effects of self-help materials, social support instructions, and telephone counseling. *J Consult Clin Psychol.* 59, 439–448.
9. Fagerström, K.O., Kunze, M. and Schoberberger, R. (1996) Nicotine dependence versus smoking prevalence: Comparison among countries and categories of smokers. *Tob Control* 5, 52–56.
10. Tucker, J.A. (1999) Changing addictive behavior: Historical and contemporary persepctives, in *Changing Addictive Behavior: Bridging Clinical and Public Health Strategies* (eds J.A. Tucker, D.A. Donovan and G.A. Marlatt), Guilford Press: New York, pp. 3–44.
11. DiClemente, C.C., Prochaska, J.O. and Gibertini M. (1985) Self-efficacy and the stages of self-change of smoking. *Cognitive Ther Res.* 9, 181–200.
12. Prochaska, J.O. and DiClemente, C.C. (eds). (1986) *Toward a Comprehensive Model of Change*, Plenum: New York.
13. Bandura, A. (1997) The anatomy of stages of change. *Am J Health Promot.* 12(1), 8–10.
14. Budd, R.J. and Rollnick, S. (1996) The structure of the Readiness to Change Questionnaire: A test of Prochaska and DiClemente's transtheoretical model. *Br J Health Psychol.* 1, 365–376.
15. Carey, K.B., Purnine, D.M., Maisto, S.A. and Carey, M.P. (1999) Assessing readiness to change substance abuse: A critical review of instruments. *Clin Psychol-Sci Pract.* 6(3), 245–266.

16. Davidson, R. (1998) The transtheoretical model: A critical overview, in *Treating Addictive Behaviors*, 2nd edn. (eds W.R. Miller and N. Heather), Plenum: New York, pp. 25–38.
17. Sutton, S. (1996) Can stages of change provide guidelines in the treatment of addictions? in *Psychotherapy, Psychological Treatments and the Addictions* (eds G. Edwards and C. Dare), Cambridge University Press: Cambridge, MA, pp. 189–205.
18. Miller, W.R. and Rollnick, S. (1991) *Motivational Interviewing: Preparing People to Change Addictive Behavior*, Guilford: New York.
19. Substance Abuse and Mental Health Administration. (1999) Enhancing motivation for change in substance abuse treatment (Treatment Improvement Protocol Series No. 35), U.S. Department of Health and Human Services: Rockville, MD.
20. Allen, J.P., Mattson, M.E., Miller, W.R. *et al.* (1997) Matching alcoholism treatments to client heterogeneity: Project MATCH posttreatment drinking outcomes. *J Stud Alcohol* **58**, 7–29.
21. Aday, L.A. and Andersen, R.M. (1974) A framework for the study of access to medical care. *Health Sci Res.* **9**, 208–220.
22. Becker, C.H. and Maiman, L.A. (1975) Sociobehavioral determinants of compliance with health and medical care recommendations. *Med Care* **13**, 10–14.
23. Thom, B. (1986) Sex differences in help-seeking for alcohol problems −1. The barriers to help-seeking. *Br J Addict.* **81**, 777–788.
24. Thom, B., Brown, C., Drummond, C., Edwards, G. and Mullan, M. (1992) The use of services for alcohol problems: General practitioner and specialist alcohol clinic. *Br J Addict.* **87**, 613–624.
25. Klingemann, H. and Hunt, G. (1998) *Drug Treatment Systems in an International Perspective*, Sage Publications Inc.: Thousand Oaks, CA.
26. Miller, W.R., Brown, J.M., Simpson, T.L. *et al.* (1995) What works? A methodological snalysis of the alcohol treatment outcome literature, in *Handbook of Alcoholism Treatment Approaches: Effective Alternatives*, 2nd edn, (eds. R.K. Hester and W.R. Miller), Allyn and Bacon: Boston, pp. 12–44.
27. Marlatt, G.A. (1999) From hindsight to foresight: A commentary on Project Match, in *Changing Addictive Behavior: Bridging Clinical and Public Health Strategies* (eds J.A. Tucker, D.A. Donovan and G.A. Marlatt), Guilford Press: New York, pp. 45–66.
28. Kavanagh, D.J., Sitharthan, T., Spilsbury, G. and Vignaedra, S. (1999) An evaluation of brief correspondence programs for problem drinkers. *Behav Ther.* **30**, 641–656.
29. Tucker, J.A. and Davison, J.W. (2000) Waiting to see the doctor: The role of time constraints in the utlization of health and behavioral health services, in *Reframing Health Behavior Change with Behavior Economics* (eds W. Bickel and R. Vuchinich), Lawrence Erlbaum: New York, pp. 219–264.
30. Pescosolido, B. (1991) Illness careers and network ties: A conceptual model of utilization and compliance. *Adv in Med Sociol.* **2**, 161–184.
31. Aasland, O.G., Bruusgaard, D. and Rutle, O. (1987) Alcohol problems in general practice. *Br J Addict.* **82**, 197–201.
32. Sobell, M.B. and Sobell, L.C. (2000) Stepped care as a heuristic approach to the treatment of alcohol problems. *J Consult Clin Psychol.* **68**, 573–579
33. Wilson, G.T. (1999) Rapid response to cognitive behavior therapy. *Clin Psychol: Sci Pract.* **6**(3), 289–292.
34. Sobell, M.B. and Sobell, L.C. (1993) Treatment for problem drinkers: A public health priority, in *Addictive Behaviors Across the Lifespan: Prevention, Treatment, and Policy Issues* (eds J.S. Baer, G.A. Marlatt and R.J. McMahon), Sage: Beverly Hills, CA, pp. 138–157.

Chapter seven

Role of minimum interventions in the natural recovery process

Given what is known about natural recovery, an inevitable question is: where do health-care providers fit in? As experts suggest, up to 82% of alcohol abusers resolve their problems without help from professionals [1]. So, why are professionals interested in getting involved? The answer, at least in part, may be because health-care providers may be able to expedite this natural, yet time-delayed, process.

To use an analogy, farmers enhance natural processes by planting in the right soil and at the right time. They know when to apply water, fertilizer, and insecticide to hasten the growth process, and they call in expert consultants when problems arise. Moreover, they know that weather conditions such as high winds or hail storms may occur that could force them to re-plant. As nurturers of a different sort of natural process, health-care providers should apply similar tactics to promote natural recovery from alcohol problems.

HOW TO BEGIN

Some health-care providers may feel unsure about when and where to intervene. The answer to that uncertainty is rather simple. Because individuals with substance abuse problems are seen in a variety of health-care settings, the time to begin is now, and the place is wherever health-care providers practice. An important thing to remember, however, is that since the natural-recovery or self-change process takes time, no one may be able to do it all, and interventions could occur at many points and in several settings. The Transtheoretical Stages of Change (TSC) model provides some direction regarding the roles that clinicians should adopt with respect to where the substance user, is in terms of readiness to change [2]. According to the TSC model, change evolves over five stages, which comprise precontemplation, contemplation, preparation, action, and maintenance. As noted in a new book on motivational interviewing [3, p. 138–139], clinicians can use a simple ruler, known as the Readiness Ruler, for determining a person's readiness to change. An example of a 'Readiness Ruler' is shown in Figure 1. Using the ruler, the clinician asks where the person is on the scale from 1 to 10. The lower the number the less ready people are to change, while higher numbers reflect more readiness to change. Because readiness to change has emerged as one of the strongest predictors of positive outcomes [4], it is suggested that it can be used along with other measures during treatment, such as self-efficacy, to identify clients who are not changing [5, 6]; at that point the intervention could be stepped up (see Chapter 6 of this book).

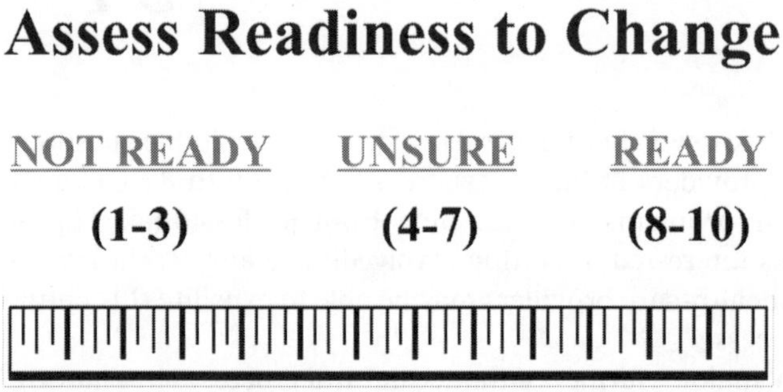

Assess Readiness to Change

NOT READY	UNSURE	READY
(1-3)	**(4-7)**	**(8-10)**

Figure 1   Readiness-to-Change Ruler.

PROMOTING SELF-CHANGE USING READINESS TO CHANGE

As shown in Table 1, it is recommended that different strategies and approaches be taken, depending on the individual's level of readiness to change. A recent and superb publication on motivational interviewing by the US Substance Abuse and Mental Health Administration [3] provides considerable clinical direction and suggestions on how to select and use various motivational interviewing strategies and techniques for substance users at different points in terms of their readiness to change. A copy of this clinical guidebook can be obtained free of cost (Contact the National Clearinghouse for Alcohol and Drug Information (NCADI) (800) 729-6686 or (301) 468–2600; TDD (for hearing impaired) (800 487–4889).

Table 1 Suggestions for what to do for clients in different stages of readiness to change

---

Clients Who Are Not Ready
- DON'T
  - Use shame and blame
  - Label, preach, stereotype or confront
  - Confront resistance

- DO
  - Provide empathic listening
  - Give feedback and show concern
  - Explore pros and cons of change
  - Negotiate: 'What would it take to consider a change?'
  - Offer information, support, and further contact

Clients Who Are Unsure
- DON'T
  - Jump ahead
  - Give advice or confront resistance
  - Expect agreement

- DO
  - Practice empathic, reflective listening (neutral, open-ended questions)
  - Explore pros and cons: 'Help me to understand through your eyes what 'x' does for you.'
  - What don't you like about your use of 'x'?'

Clients Who Are Ready
- DON'T jump in with simple advice

- EXPLORE pros and cons of treatment

- DO EMPHASIZE
  - Alternatives (community resources)
  - Known role models
  - Autonomy ('You are the best judge')
  - Choice ('What will work for you?')
  - Optimism ('Treatment works')
  - Back-up ('If this doesn't work, call me')

Not thinking of changing

During the early stages of change individuals are generally unaware of their problems and have no intention of changing in the foreseeable future.

Interestingly, despite people's personal lack of insight others whom they know (e.g. relatives, friends, employers, legal authorities, health-care providers) often recognize that they have a problem.

50-Year Old Naturally Recovered Male Describing The Early Stages Of His Drinking Problem

'I just fell into the habit of drinking beer every day. I might only drink two or three every evening or sometimes it might be six or eight or twelve. It wasn't to get drunk, it was just a habit'.

Insight From a Significant Other

'My mom wouldn't let me play rugby because of my drinking. I really valued being on the team. It was one of the most important things in my life. But the threat of not being able to play didn't keep me from drinking'.

Individuals who engage in treatment while they are not yet ready often do so because of pressure from others. Once this pressure abates or they are outside a structured treatment setting, people in the precontemplation stage usually revert to old habits [2].

As individuals move from the stage of not thinking about it to that of just thinking about it, they acknowledge that a problem exists and begin to consider overcoming it.

Thinking About It

'There was a period of time between marriages when I was aware that I was drinking more than I should. I wasn't really frightened by it, I just knew I was doing it. I actually wrote some fairly lengthy letters to a friend about it'.

Although individuals in this stage have become somewhat aware of their problems, they have not made a firm commitment to change. One of the features of this stage is that individuals weigh the pros and cons of their alcohol abuse and begin to formulate solutions to their problems [1, 2].

Starting To Evaluate the Negative Aspects of Drinking

'There was a sense of fear about what I was doing to myself, what I had lost, or what I might see myself losing. I don't think it was quite so much a physical fear yet, except that I was really worried about memory blackouts. That frightened me a lot. I guess I was facing the possibility that I was doing things to myself that would make it impossible to be what I wanted to be'.

In the early stages of change or readiness to change, the challenge to health-care providers is to hasten their progression. In terms of the agricultural analogy used earlier, the question becomes what kind of fertilizers and pesticides should be used to speed up the natural recovery process? According to Prochaska et al. [2] individuals in the precontemplation and contemplation stages are most amenable to consciousness-raising activities such as information gathering, self-observation, and emotive experiences. In addition, the importance of empowering people by promoting their self-efficacy (i.e. perception of personal capability) cannot be overemphasized, since individuals will not take steps to improve their situations if they believe they are helpless and their conditions are hopeless [7].

To raise self-awareness and self-efficacy, it has been suggested that health-care providers share information with individuals about their substance use by discussing the results of a substance use assessment [2]. Specific feedback or advice can be given to clients about their past use (for examples of such feedback and how it should be used, see [3, 8]). Such advice can enhance or strengthen motivation for change [8–11]. In fact, such an assessment has reduced alcohol use by 20% among clients in primary-care settings [12]. By heightening clients' awareness in this manner, it is thought that they are at least partially empowered to work independently through the stages of change.

Needless to say, allowing clients in early stages of readiness to change to work at their own pace may be difficult for some service providers who are accustomed to employing highly structured treatment programs. This may be especially true if individuals fail to act promptly on information. Indeed, some clients may need to be exposed to the same basic information several times before they move past these early stages of change.

To complicate matters, the most appropriate dosing and timing of advice and feedback may be unique for each individual and highly dependent upon subjective factors that are difficult to assess. Lacking a predictable time line, it is still important for health-care providers to inform and advise clients about their risky behavior in order to promote self-change. For examples of alcohol use advice and feedback, readers are referred to two publications [3, 8, pp. 69–70] as well as the Self-Change Toolbox, in the Appendix to this book.

Preparation stage

Within the preparation or decision-making stage, intention and behavior begin to coalesce. Clients may have reached this stage if health-care providers readily hold their attention when discussing their alcohol use, drug use or smoking. In addition, clients may begin to ask questions or they may share their preliminary attempts to change.

Preparing to Change

'I started to moderate over a couple of years. I probably cut it back to getting severely drunk only once a week instead of twice or sometimes 4 or 5 times a week'.

Individuals may also talk about substituting new activities to change their substance abuse or altering their environments to avoid substance-related triggers.

Substituting New Activities

To fill time that would normally be reserved for drinking, an individual explained, 'I started walking, watching educational television, going to the library and reading voraciously about race relations, and painting'.

Finally, clients may look for indications from clinicians that their situation is not hopeless, and that they have the power to make things better for themselves independently [13].

Efforts to promote self-change may be aided by emphasizing that a large number of people resolve an alcohol, drug or nicotine problem with little or no professional intervention [13, 14]. It may also be therapeutic for both client and health-care provider to review the temporal nature of change so that overly enthusiastic expectations are not dashed by the amount of time that may be necessary for individuals to fully enter the action stage. Finally, during the early stages of change it is important to remain nonjudgmental. In this regard, a motivational interviewing approach which is designed to deal with ambivalent individuals can accomplish this objective [3].

Action stage

The action stage of change is exciting as committed individuals alter their drinking habits and visible improvements in their behavior are evident.

Committed to Change

'Before, I wouldn't want to go out with my wife because I'd had a few beers. I didn't want to get out and drive. After I quit drinking, it was a new life'.

During this stage, clients may look for support from peers and significant others. Self-changers may also continue to be eager for input from professionals. Thus, this is a good time to share specific self-change strategies that will continue to promote empowerment and instill hope [13].

Spousal Support

My husband knew when I wanted to drink. He and I were that in tune. He'd say, 'It's okay. Let's deal with this. Let's talk about this. Do you need some space? Drinking is not going to make this any better'".

During this time, relapses or slips are likely to be encountered.

Lapse/Slip: What Do I Do?

'I was 3 hours away from home, and everybody up there drank. It wasn't as bad as the time before, but I started drinking. And pretty soon, whooops! I had to back off. It was no where near as bad as the first time'.

Across all addictive behavior relapse is a serious problem. The highest relapse rate occurs within the first three to six months following treatment [15–17]. In light of such figures, professionals have not always looked realistically at the possibility that clients will make progress toward resolving their substance use problems while still experiencing periodic setbacks. Prochaska *et al.* [2] view this process of spiraling in and out as normal, and the harm reduction literature offers a framework for viewing any small steps in the right direction as successes [20]. Indeed, it has been suggested that the real test of change is long-term sustained change over many years [9, 19].

Another mistake that health-care providers may make as the action stage begins to emerge is to become overly controlling. That is, since clients have demonstrated a tendency toward change, some clinicians may assume that they are enthusiastic about receiving highly structured assistance in the form of traditional inpatient or outpatient services. Thus, for individuals who have come to health-care professionals with hopes of changing their problems on their own, relegating them to the sick-person role may be counterproductive [3]. Motivational interviewing suggests taking a nonjudgmental, nonconfrontational, nonlabelling approach to all clients [3]. Lastly, the literature suggests taking a stepped-care approach to treatment – that is, one that considers the least restrictive, least intrusive, least costly, and most consumer-appealing intervention available [20, 21].

Self-guided change resources

There are a number of ways in which clients can be empowered to help themselves during the action stage. Self-change guide-books are available in book stores [22], and one testimony to the profound need for such resources is that some of them are being written by individuals at the grassroots level [23]. Examples of such books and where to get them are provided in the Self-Change Toolbox of this book.

Individuals who are lucky enough to find an enlightened practitioner can be guided through a self-help process that involves setting personalized goals, monitoring their own drinking triggers and habits, and independently making decisions. In these instances, professionals are largely responsible for initiating the process, answering technical questions, and serving as sounding boards [26].

Another resource for individuals who are pursuing a self-help approach is the World-Wide Web. Sites such as HabitSmart < www.cts.com/crash/habtsmrt > provide a broad range of self-help information. In addition, online groups such as the Moderation Management[T] listserv <http://moderation.org/index. html> offer peer support 24 hours a day. It is important for health-care providers to be aware of these types of resources and to screen them for their relevancy and efficacy. This is particularly important in light of their low cost, providing individuals have access to a computer. The Appendix contains several useful websites and self-guided resources.

Maintenance stage

Resources such as online support groups may prove to be particularly helpful for individuals who have experienced the elation of taking action and want to continue to maintain that change. These individuals may simply need the friendship and support that peers with similar problems can continue to provide. As such, easily accessible, affordable, and nonstigmatizing online resources may once again be particularly helpful since individuals can access them on an 'as needed' basis for months or years to come. In fact, social support is one of the most important factors associated with positive sustained outcomes with or without treatment [1, 19, 25]. In summary, maintenance is best conceptualized, not as an absence of change, but rather as the continuance of change [26].

INSTITUTING NATURAL RECOVERY TREATMENT STRATEGIES

Implementing new self-change treatment strategies in clinical settings may be somewhat challenging for some clinicians owing to a variety of factors. First, old mind-sets are difficult to change, and many health-care providers are comfortable using the traditional more-is-better treatment approach. Other challenges range from pragmatic clinical concerns to financial issues.

Financial concerns

In relationship to financial concern, if recovery from substance use problems occurs naturally (or with limited professional intervention), some clinicians may worry about the security of their jobs. Further, if substance abuse problems can be self-resolved, why should clinicians be reimbursed for treating them? That is, private and governmental health-care agencies are in the business of paying for treatment of diseases, not bad habits. However, because many individuals never cross the clinical threshold to enter treatment programs or go to self-help meetings, it is unlikely that the field is going to run out of individuals who are in need of services.

The disease paradigm of alcohol abuse has also been promoted by the pharmaceutical industry, which gets profits by treating diseases. Moreover, drug companies have marketing departments and sales people that sell their products to health-care providers and the general public. As such, little time or cost is required for health-care providers to prescribe a cure in a capsule (e.g. anti-depressants) versus helping clients work through the self-change process.

Need for clinicians to re-tool

Helping clients work through the self-change process on their own may take some re-tooling on the part of many mental health-care professions who are accustomed to the old one-size-fits-all-approach [20, 21]. Using the concept of 'readiness to change,' clinicians are asked to view clients as individuals who are at different places on the continuum of change [3]. They are also asked to accept that not everyone will readily respond to a single intervention and to use the tools of motivational interviewing to promote commitment to change by considering where the client is in the change process. The recent Motivational Interviewing volume in the Treatment Improvement Protocol (TIP) Series suggests that a broad range of assessment and intervention skills is needed to effectively assist clients through all phases of the change process [3]. This volume contains the following useful information for health-care practitioners working with substance abusers, including over a dozen screening and assessment instruments and other resources along with how to use and obtain such information.

Broadening the base of interventionists

An unsettling notion to some may be that the wrong group of health-care providers has been targeted to promote the self-change process. That is, although psychiatrists, psychologists, and social workers play a crucial role in treating alcohol abuse, many times they are not the first to recognize that clients are experiencing problems related to their drinking. Rather, health-care providers in family practice settings are much more likely to be the first to notice early warning signs. This has to do with the fact that practitioners in these settings normally see clients more often than other types of clinicians. Further, primary-care providers frequently serve as gatekeepers to other services such as mental health care.

Unfortunately, health-care providers in family practice settings have yet to be given many practical tools to use to promote the natural recovery process. A clear illustration is the dearth of short assessment instruments (i.e. 1 or 2 questions) to diagnose mild to moderate alcohol problems. That is, considering the number of other crucial areas that practitioners must assess as part of a general screening exam, lengthy diagnostic protocols are impractical. The assessment instrument should also be user friendly, free, consumer appealing, easy to score, and be able to provide advice and feedback to individuals to help increase their motivation to change [3, 10, 11, 27]. On an optimistic note, three studies show that a single question about alcohol use may prove to be effective in screening/recognizing at-risk drinkers [28–30].

Another problem is that, although researchers have demonstrated the efficacy of brief interventions in family practice settings [31, 32], their effectiveness has not been confirmed. The distinction made here is that, for the most part, brief interventions have been tested under optimum conditions rather than in real-world primary health-care settings [33]. In short, the crucial need is to test very brief (i.e. a few minutes) interventions on the part of regular clinic staff under routine office conditions.

Other health-care settings that offer opportunities for clinicians to provide brief interventions are inpatient medical/surgical wards and emergency rooms [33]. Although few patients come to these settings primarily for the treatment of alcohol abuse disorders, many times it is clear to health-care providers that drinking is an underlying problem. In the past, clinicians have not taken advantage of these opportunities to intervene because they were steeped in the long-term alcohol treatment paradigm and were unconvinced that their efforts would be effective. As more evidence dispels this belief, hospital-based practitioners should make brief interventions part of their routine care.

CONCLUSIONS AND FUTURE DIRECTIONS

Getting the message out: dissemination

Another barrier that has prevented the rapid acceptance of brief interventions has been the tendency of researchers to preach to the converted. That is, scholarly research reports have their merit, but many front-line practitioners do not read this literature and are not prepared to readily understand it and infer sound clinical interventions [34]. This is also true in the drug addiction field, where clinical workers may not be professionally trained in psychology, nursing, social work, or medicine. Moreover, many of those who have been trained to work with alcohol abusers have not been exposed to natural-recovery precepts, since most textbooks do not include this information.

Borrowing from the sales departments of pharmaceutical companies, Sobell [34] has argued that if researchers want brief intervention strategies to become common practice, they should market their product better. In other words, researchers should consider developing an evidence-based treatment package that can be sold in a five-minute sales pitch. Moreover, introductory materials such as self-help guides should be left in health-care facilities for clinicians to review, just as free drug samples are made available for health-care providers to use on a trial basis.

Educating the general public

Results from several studies across multiple addictions [reviewed in 14, 19, 35–38] reveal that self-change is a major pathway to recovery. Unfortunately, however, most people are not aware of this fact [39, 40]. One reason is that the media continue to perpetuate the concept of substance abuse as a disease requiring treatment. Thus, to overcome this wrong impression the public's awareness about self-change as a way of recovering from alcohol problems needs to be heightened. For example, campaigns should be mounted to educate the general public about the self-change process. Also, informing health-care practitioners about the viability of self-change or assisted self-change could help them feel more comfortable with this approach so that they can converse with their clients from an informed viewpoint.

REFERENCES

1. Sobell, L.C., Sobell, M.B., Toneatto, T. and Leo, G.I. (1993) What triggers the resolution of alcohol problems without treatment? *Alcohol: Clin Exp Res.* **17**(2), 217–224.
2. Prochaska, J.O., Norcross, J.C. and DiClemente, C.C. (1994) *Changing for Good: A Revolutionary Six-Stage Program for Ovecoming Bad Habits and Moving your Life Positively Forward*, Avon Books: New York.
3. Substance Abuse and Mental Health Administration. (1999) Enhancing motivation for change in substance abuse treatment (Treatment Improvement Protocol Series No. 35). U.S. Department of Health and Human Services: Rockville, MD.
4. Project MATCH Research Group. (1998) Matching alcoholism treatments to client heterogeneity: Project MATCH three-year drinking outcomes. *Alcohol: Clin Exp Res.* **22**, 1300–1311.
5. Breslin, F.C., Sobell, M.B., Sobell, L.C., Buchan, G. and Cunningham, J.A. (1997) Toward a stepped care approach to treating problem drinkers: The predictive utility of within-treatment variables and therapist prognostic ratings. *Addiction* **92**(11), 1479–1489.
6. Breslin, F.C., Sobell, M.B., Sobell, L.C., Cunningham, J.A., Sdao-Jarvie, K. and Borsoi, D. (1999) Problem drinkers: Evaluation of a stepped care approach. *J Subst Abuse* **10**, 217–232.
7. Bandura, A. (1997) *Self-Efficacy: The Exercise of Control*, W.H. Freeman: New York.
8. Sobell, L.C., Cunningham, J.C., Sobell, M.B. *et al.* (1996) Fostering self-change among problem drinkers: A proactive community intervention. *Addict Behav.* **21**(6), 817–833.
9. Miller, W.R. and Rollnick, S. (1991) *Motivational Interviewing: Preparing People to Change Addictive Behavior*, Guilford: New York.
10. Sobell, L.C. and Sobell, M.B. (1998) Identification and assessment of alcohol problems, in *Psychologist's Desk Reference* (eds G.P. Koocher, J.A. Norcross and S.S. Hill), Oxford University Press: New York, pp. 62–67.
11. Sobell, L.C. and Sobell, M.B. (2000) Drug abuse, in *Encyclopedia of Psychology* (ed. A.E. Kazdin), American Psychological Association and Oxford University Press: New York and Washington, DC, pp. 93–97.
12. Fleming, M.F., Barry, K.L., Manwell, L.B., Johnson, K. and London, R. (1997) Brief physician advice for problem alcohol drinkers: A rendomized controlled trial in community-based primary care practices. *JAMA.* **277**, 1039–1045.
13. Finfgeld, D.L. (1999) Use of brief interventions to treat individuals with drinking problems. *J Psychosoc Nurs Ment Health Serv.* **37**(4), 23–30.
14. Sobell, L.C., Cunningham, J.A. and Sobell, M.B. (1996) Recovery from alcohol problems with and without treatment: Prevalence in two population surveys. *Am J Public Health* **86**(7), 966–972.
15. Allsop, S., Saunders, B., Phillips, M. and Carr, A. (1997) A trial of relapse prevention with severely dependent male problem drinkers. *Addiction* **92**, 61–73.
16. Hunt, W.A., Barnett, L.W. and Branch, L.G. (1971) Relapse rates in addiction programs. *J Clin Psychol.* **27**, 455–456.
17. Marlatt, G.A. and Gordon, J.R. (1985) *Relapse Prevention*, Guilford Press: New York.

18. Marlatt, G.A. (1998) *Harm Reduction: Pragmatic Strategies for Managing High-Risk Behaviors*, Guilford Press: New York.
19. Sobell, L.C., Ellingstad, T.P. and Sobell, M.B. (2000) Natural recovery from alcohol and drug problems: Methodological review of the research with suggestions for future directions. *Addiction* **95**, 749–769.
20. Sobell, M.B. and Sobell, L.C. (2000) Stepped care as a heuristic approach to the treatment of alcohol problems. *J Consult Clin Psychol.* **68**, 573–579.
21. Sobell, M.B. and Sobell, L.C. (1999) Stepped care for alcohol problems, An efficient method for planning and delivering clinical services, in *Changing Addictive Behavior: Bridging Clinical and Public Health Strategies* (eds J.A. Tucker, D.A. Donovan and G.A. Marlatt), Guilford Press: New York, pp. 331–343.
22. Horvath, A.T. (1998) Sex, drugs, gambling and chocolate: A workbook for overcoming addictions, Impact: San Luis, Opispo, CA.
23. Kishline, A. (1994) *Moderate Drinking: The Moderation Management Guide for People who Want to Reduce their Drinking*, Crown Trade Paperbacks: New York.
24. Sobell, M.B. and Sobell, L.C. (1993) *Problem Drinkers: Guided Self-Change Treatment*, Guilford Press: New York.
25. Sobell, M.B., Sobell, L.C. and Leo, G.I. (2000) Does enhanced social support improve outcomes for problem drinkers in Guided Self-Change treatment. *J Behav Ther Exp Psychiatry.* **31**, 41–54
26. Prochaska, J.O. and DiClemente, C.C. (eds) (1986) Toward a comprehensive model of change, in *Treating Addictive Behaviors: Processes of Change* (eds W.E. Miller and N. Heather), Plenum: New York, pp. 3–27.
27. Sobell, M.B., Agrawal, S., Leo, G.I., Young-Johnson, L., Sobell. M.B. and Cunningham, J.C. (1999) Quick drinking screen versus the alcohol Timeline Followback: A time and place for both procedures, in *Poster Presented at the 33rd Annual Meeting of the Association for Advancement of Behavior Therapy*, November 1999, Toronto, Ontario, Canada.
28. Cyr, M.G. and Wartman, S.A. (1988) The effectiveness of routine screening questions in the detection of alcoholism. *JAMA.* **259**, 51–54.
29. Woodruff, R.A., Clayton, P.J., Cloninger. R. and Guze, S.B. (1976) A brief method of screening for alcoholism. *Dis Nerv Syst.* **37**, 434–435.
30. Taj, N., Devera-Sales, A. and Vinson, D.C. (1998) Screening for problem drinking: Does a single question work? *J Fam Pract.* **46**, 328–335.
31. Fleming, M. and Manwell, L.B. (1999) Brief intervention in primary care settings: A primary treatment method for at-risk, problem, and dependent drinkers. *Alcohol Health Res. World* **23**(2), 128–137.
32. Fleming, M.F., Manwell, L.B., Barry, K.L., Adams, W. and Stauffacher, E.A. (1999) Brief physician advice for alcohol problems in older adults: A randomized community-based trial. *J Fam Pract.* **48**, 378–384.
33. Heather, N. (1998) Using brief opportunities for change in medical settings, in *Treating Addictive Behaviors* (eds W.R. Miller and N. Heather), Plenum: New York, pp. 133–147.
34. Sobell, L.C. (1996) Bridging the gap between scientists and practitioners: The challenge before us. *Behav Ther.* **27**(3), 297–320.
35. Hodgins, D.C., Wynne, H. and Makarchuk, K. (1999) Pathways to recovery from gambling problems: Follow-up from a general population survey. *J Gambling Stud.* **15**, 93–104.
36. Hodgins, D.C. and El-Guebaly, N. (2000) Natural and treatment-assisted recovery from gambling problems: A comparison of resolved and active gamblers. *Addiction* **95**, 777–789.
37. Fiore, M.C., Novotny, T.E., Pierce, J.P. *et al.* (1990) Methods used to quit smoking in the United States. *JAMA.* **263**, 2760–2765.

38. Orleans, C.T., Schoenbach, V.J., Wagner, E.H. *et al.* (1991) Self-help quit smoking interventions: Effects of self-help materials, social support instructions, and telephone counseling. *J Consult Clin Psychol.* **59**, 439–448.
39. Cunningham, J.A., Sobell, L.C. and Sobell, M.B. (1998) Awareness of self-change as a pathway to recovery for alcohol abusers: Results from five different groups. *Addict Behav.* **23**(3), 399–404.
40. Cunningham, J.A., Sobell, L.C. and Chow, V.M.C. (1993) What's in a label? The effects of substance types and labels on treatment considerations and stigma. *J Stud Alcohol* **54**, 693–699.

Chapter eight

Taking the treatment to the community

As discussed in Chapter 1, because the vast majority of substance abusers are unlikely to enter traditional substance abuse treatment programs there is a serious need to develop and evaluate alternative, minimally intrusive interventions that appeal to individuals with substance use problems. If substance users are unwilling to come into treatment, what can be done to motivate them to change their substance use?

Over the past decade procedures to increase motivation have become a common feature of many cognitive-behavioral interventions with alcohol and other drug abusers [1]. Motivation has been conceptualized as a state that is changeable and reflects various features of a person's history and the presenting situation [1, 2]. As part of his general cognitive social learning theory of behavior, Bandura also discusses variables that can affect motivation [3]. Motivation can be enhanced in several ways: (a) providing advice and feedback; (b) removing barriers to change; (c) allowing people as much perceived choice of interventions as possible; (d) decreasing the attractiveness of substance use; (e) arranging external contingencies to encourage and support change; (f) providing personal feedback about the effects of problem behavior (e.g. alcohol, drug, and cigarette use, gambling) as a way of reinforcing change; (g) setting clear and feasible goals; and (h) expressing a helping attitude [1, 2].

If people will not cross the clinical threshold or come into treatment, it has been proposed to 'take the treatment' to the people [4]. That is, rather than providing treatment at traditional substance abuse agencies, interventions could be provided in non-traditional settings such as over the internet or by mail. Efficient methods of promoting self-change in community settings would allow widespread impact on substance use problems and, if successful, at a much lower cost than traditional outpatient services.

137

SELF-CHANGE APPROACHES

Self-change approaches have long been part of many brief interventions that help substance abusers evaluate and guide their own behavior change [5–10]. Factors associated with the development of self-change approaches include: (1) the need for interventions for persons whose substance abuse problems are not severe, particularly those with alcohol problems [9–11]; (2) demonstrations that for many individuals brief interventions are as beneficial as more intense interventions [12–16]; and (3) an emphasis on self-control processes in the evolution of cognitive-behavior therapy [17, 18].

The success of brief self-change treatment for substance abusers suggests that even before entering treatment such individuals possess sufficient skills to function effectively [19]. This, in turn, suggests that the major function of such treatment might be motivational – to catalyze individuals' use of their own resources to bring about behavior change. In a study that provides some support for the idea that self-change approaches and minimal interventions might appeal to adult drinkers, Werch [20] found that over one quarter of all drinkers reported an interest in receiving aids to help them drink more moderately. Moreover, drinkers who were interested in receiving one or more self-help aids reported high levels of drinking and a greater motivation to limit their alcohol use. This study suggests that a considerable number of drinkers, especially heavier drinkers, would be receptive to aids to help them drink less.

A non-traditional way of facilitating self-change with regard to excessive drinking has been through the use of very brief interventions by physicians in primary care health settings. These interventions usually consist of a brief inquiry followed by brief advice if warranted. An important characteristic of these interventions is that typically the patients' reasons for seeing their physician have nothing to do with drinking. However, as part of the visit the physician inquires about alcohol use and if the patient's drinking exceeds recommended guidelines [21] the physician raises that issue and suggests the patient reduce his or her drinking to recommended levels. Such interventions have produced significant decreases in drinking and can reach a much broader population than that served by substance abuse programs [5].

Another approach that would be considered a minimal intervention in terms of necessary time and resource expenditure and that also allows access to geographically difficult-to-reach populations is intervention by correspondence or by telephone [8, 22–26].

The utility of a correspondence version of a brief self-change approach for use in rural communities was demonstrated in a recent study [8]. This study, which evaluated a 4-month intervention delivered by correspondence for 121 problem drinkers recruited by media advertisements, compared a cognitive-behavioral (CBT) intervention with a minimal intervention (e.g. educational material and suggestions to self-monitor drinking). As predicted, CBT was more effective than MI in reducing alcohol consumption over the 4-month intervention (i.e. CBT produced a 50% fall in consumption, bringing the average intake of individuals to less than recommended maximum levels). Treatment gains at 6 months were maintained at 12 months, despite the MI group being given the CBT materials at 4 months. High levels of consumer satisfaction, a high representation of women and substantial participation from isolated rural areas attested to the feasibility of the correspondence program as an alternative treatment. The results supported the use of correspondence delivery as a means of promoting early engagement and equity of access between city and country areas.

Another tactic that can be used for community level interventions is media campaigns. Several studies have evaluated the value of media campaigns for reducing the prevalence of smoking and reported positive effects [27–35]. Often these campaigns involve large-scale advertising either about the health risks of smoking or deriding the positive symbolic value of smoking behavior (e.g. it's not cool to smoke). Interestingly, large community intervention trials or mass media campaigns aimed at secondary prevention have focused almost exclusively on cigarette use. Such campaigns for other addictive behavior (e.g. gambling, alcohol or drug problems), with one exception [4], have been lacking. Finally, another new and promising way of accessing the community on a large scale is through the Internet [36, 37]. Readers interested in a further discussion of the Internet as a possible intervention strategy should see Chapter 5 of this volume.

In a review of brief interventions, Heather [38] concluded: 'Evidence shows that brief interventions are effective and should be used for individuals who are not actively seeking help at specialist agencies. This justification is, again independent of level of seriousness, although most recipients of community-based interventions will obviously have problems of a less severe variety' (p. 366).

A COMMUNITY DEMONSTRATION: BACKGROUND AND RATIONALE

The Fostering Self-Change (FSC) project, a community level intervention, funded through the National Institute of Alcohol Abuse and Alcoholism, is being conducting in Canada [4]. This large-scale community intervention was designed to promote or foster self-change among individuals who were unwilling, not ready, or otherwise unmotivated to access the formal health care system in order to change their drinking. As will be discussed later, while the FSC intervention was designed for problem drinkers, several aspects of the project are relevant to prevention and harm reduction. For example, avenues and procedures that will attract individuals in the general public to consider changing their drinking on their own or with minimal help are likely to be very different from what traditional practices in the alcohol field would suggest. Finally, while the FSC community trial was designed for problem drinkers, coupled with the fact, as noted above, that community interventions are successful with cigarette smokers, there is every reason to extend and evaluate such trials to individuals with other types of addictive behavior.

The FSC intervention represents a convergence of two lines of research. The first involved studies that examined the natural recovery processes with alcohol abusers [39, 40], and the second involved clinical trials using a Guided Self-Change model of treatment with problem drinkers [9, 19]. This community-based intervention was designed to take account of three factors found to be associated with heavy drinkers who do not seek formal help or treatment [reviewed in 4]: (a) stigma or embarrassment of being in treatment for alcohol problems; (b) the desire to change on one's own; and (c) little belief by the general public that self-change is a viable pathway to recovery.

Designed to increase the prevalence of recovery in the community without using formal help or treatment, the FSC project took elements from the Guided Self-Change treatment procedures (e.g. Decisional Balance Exercise, Brief Situational Confidence Questionnaire, Timeline Drinking Advice/Feedback [9, 19]) and made them available by mail to individuals in the community who wanted to change their drinking on their own.

The conceptual framework upon which the FSC intervention was based will be briefly discussed. Self-change approaches, of which the current intervention is one, are designed to help problem drinkers analyse their own problems and guide their own change. Factors associated with the development of the FSC intervention are the same as those discussed for self-change approaches.

BRIEF DESCRIPTION OF THE FSC PROJECT

Individuals volunteered for the FSC project by responding to media solicitations and if eligible were sent assessment materials. After the materials were completed and returned by mail, the respondents in the experimental condition were sent a set of personalized feedback materials relating to their drinking levels, high-risk situations, and motivation to change (see Appendix A4). Respondents assigned to the control group were sent two educational pamphlets rather than personalized feedback. The sample consisted of 825 respondents recruited primarily through newspaper advertisements that stated: 'Thinking about changing your drinking? Do you know that 75% of people change their drinking on their own. Call for free mail out materials.' If this minimal-intensity mailed-out intervention were successful the intervention would allow large numbers of people to be served at a relatively low cost. The advertisements resulted in an unexpectedly large number of inquiries – close to 2500 people called in response.

In terms of study criteria, eligible respondents had to be of legal drinking age (i.e. 19 years in Ontario, Canada). Callers were screened by phone for a history of previous alcohol treatment or help. Excluding people with a prior history of treatment helped to ensure that severely dependent alcohol abusers were not included in a brief intervention. Eligible respondents had to report drinking an average of > 12 drinks per week or having consumed 5 or more drinks on 5 days in the past year.

Of the 2434 individuals who responded to the media solicitations for the FSC project, almost three-quarters (72%) met the initial screening criteria and were sent a consent form and the assessment questionnaires. The major reasons respondents were deemed ineligible for the intervention were that (a) 90% reported that they had previously received some type of treatment or help; and (b) 7% were ineligible because of the drinking criteria (i.e. their drinking was not heavy enough to meet the study criteria). Of those that met the initial screening criteria and were mailed out assessment packages, 47% (825 individuals) returned their questionnaires and were randomly assigned to one of the two groups. One-third of the participants were women and there were no gender differences in terms of the screening criteria.

TAILORED NON-TRADITIONAL MESSAGES IN THE FSC PROJECT

Several studies have shown that the overwhelming reason that people give for either not entering or delaying entering treatment is the stigma associated with being labeled [41–44].

Recovered Alcohol Abuser

'You are an alcoholic.' People had suggested it to me before but I never really – I had vehemently denied the idea you know or the accusation.'

In the substance abuse field, if we are to develop programs and messages that are perceived as attractive and listened to rather than avoided, then it will be necessary to understand why many individuals, even with minimal alcohol and drug problems, do not seek treatment. What this tells us is that such labels as 'alcoholic' and 'drug addict' or 'alcohol abuser' should be avoided. Such negative messages are likely to be perceived as inaccurate by high-risk drinkers in the general population. Consistent with the literature, highly effective messages will avoid stigmatizing or labeling. Second, the message needs to be proactive. Third, the message should contain information that allows people to make better and informed decisions about how much they should drink.

Over the years, whether in Canada, Australia, the USA, Sweden or Mexico, studies have recruited alcohol and drug abusers to treatment with carefully worded statements to attract such individuals. The ads for treatment typically say such things as 'Are you concerned about your alcohol or drug use?' or 'Are you considering changing your drinking?' [19, 45–48].

Recovered Alcohol Abusers Answers to the Question:

'If an ad were to appear on television or in a newspaper to attract individuals to seek help with their drinking problem what wording would you suggest'?

Respondent 1: 'If you could say something I guess maybe to indicate something like 'You can do it.' 'Help yourself, you can do it.' Something to give them some assurance that all is not lost.'

Respondent 2: 'Well, that's an interesting question. I would say something that would offer some comfort and dignity to the listener. The words that come to my mind, 'Are you sure'?

Respondent 3: 'People who drink too much are done a disservice by the use of the word alcoholic.'

Respondent 4: 'I would say more along the lines of getting people to realize they have a problem. Something like 'Do you drink every day? If you do, you may have a problem.' A non-threatening thing that would say, that somebody might say 'You know I do drink every day' and then they might make a concerted effort to not drink every day. Something very very simple. Not going into the blackouts and all. It's non-threatening. Just saying 'Do you drink every day?' Not using scare tactics, just using the tactics of be aware.'

In many ways, attempting to persuade high-risk drinkers to reduce their drinking can be approached as an exercise in attitude change. Research in cognitive social psychology tells us that when people receive a message with which they disagree they resist it by various means, such as formulating counter-arguments [49]. For example, if people who are high-risk drinkers are told 'You are an alcoholic' or 'You have an alcohol problem', they are likely to generate reasons why they are not. The message does not make sense to them. The way to avoid such counter-arguments is to present the message in a nonconfrontational and nonthreatening manner, the same strategy as used in motivational interviewing in clinical situations [1]. What we know from recruiting problem drinkers into treatment as well as getting people to respond to advertisements about changing their drinking on their own is that the 'content' of the message is critical in terms of whether people respond.

Recovered Alcohol Abuser

'So the desire is gone and this is where I part company with Alcoholics Anonymous and people like them, because they operate on a naturalistic bias. A naturalistic way whereas not necessarily Alcoholics Anonymous, because AA started as a Christian organization. But they say you are always an alcoholic.'

Because the substance abuse field has long been dominated by an almost exclusive focus on individuals who are severely dependent on alcohol, the general public, particularly in North America, has developed a stereotypic and stigmatizing impression of *anyone* who might consider reducing their drinking – such individuals are viewed as 'alcoholic' or at the very least as having an alcohol problem. It is no surprise then that trying to persuade substance abusers in the general population, whose use might be placing them at risk, to change is difficult at best, and impossible, at worst.

With respect to prevention and harm reduction, the same reasoning underlying motivational interventions can be used with the general public [50, 51]. Hhow messages are presented and what those messages say is probably even more important with substance users in the general population than self-identified problem users who are considering changing. The reason is that substance abusers in the general public are not apt to perceive themselves as needing to change. Thus, they are likely to be more resistant to messages suggesting change than would be substance abusers who are already ambivalent about their alcohol or drug use.

For a message to be considered by, and have an impact on, an individual it is important that the message does not evoke resistance. For example, because a small amount of drinking can have a cardiovascular protective effect [52, 53], a proactive prevention message could be created about the beneficial effects of limited drinking, but emphasizing that with drinking, like so many other aspects of our lives, there needs to be a healthy balance between what one gets out of drinking and the risks that are taken. A proactive message is less likely to evoke resistance than a critical message.

In summary, what the results of early intervention trials suggest for prevention and harm reduction efforts is that it will be very important to create a message, and a system for delivering that message, that is welcomed by substance users and abusers. The message cannot evoke resistance or it will be ignored and thus be ineffective. An effective strategy, however, can deliver a message that will be viewed as personally relevant and convincing. Several studies have also suggested that tailored messages may be more effective with certain groups of people [54–56]. Lastly, clinicians and researchers 'need to be sensitive to issues of stigma and disenfranchisement and to the social context of consumers' lives.'

The advertisement for the FSC project contained three messages and all were chosen to address issues or concerns we had anticipated in recruiting a group of heavy drinkers who had never accessed the health care system for their drinking. A copy of this advertisement appears in the box below. The first line of the ad: 'Thinking of Changing Your Drinking?' was chosen because it was felt that this message would not evoke resistance and would get people to think about their drinking, and for those already thinking about changing might heighten their motivation to change. The second line read 'Did you know that 75% of people change their drinking on their own'? The reason for this message was that though some Canadian studies [57, 58] had shown that over 75% of individuals with an alcohol problem change their drinking without formal treatment or AA, the general public is either skeptical about or does not believe that someone can change on their own [42, 59, 60]. Further, this message clearly puts forth the concept of empowerment [61]. The third message 'Call us for free materials that can be completed at home' was chosen because one of the major reasons that people have given for not entering treatment was that they wanted to change their drinking on their own [40, 62]. In summary, the message we were trying to communicate was that self-change was possible, asserting that over 75% of individuals change their drinking on their own.

About two-thirds of the way through the study it was decided to ask all remaining callers ($n = 605$) an open-ended question about what attracted them to the advertisements (multiple response were coded): (a) 29.4% ($n = 178$) said it was the title of the ad – 'Thinking about changing your drinking'; (b) 27.4% ($n = 166$) said it was the statement that '75% of people changed on their own'; (c) 12.9% (78) said they wanted to change at home and didn't want to come into treatment; (d) 12.1% ($n = 73$) said they just saw the ad and called; (e) 3.8% (23) said the sponsorship by the 'University of Toronto/Addiction Research Foundation'; (f) 1.7% (10) said that they responded because of the 'free materials' offered; and (g) 1.7% ($n = 10$) said it was because of the promise of 'confidentiality.' Obviously, the statements of 'Thinking of Changing Your Drinking' as well as learning that the vast majority of individuals with alcohol problems change on their own were messages that were attention-getting and effective in getting problem drinkers to call for further information.

Thinking About Changing Your Drinking?

Did you know that 75% of people change their drinking on their own? CALL US for free materials you can complete at home. (416) 595-6071. All calls are confidential. Sponsored by the University of Toronto and the Addiction Research Foundation.

ATTITUDE CHANGE

Recovered Alcohol Abuser

'Well, as I mentioned previously I had tried to stop on several occasions previously and I would stop maybe for a short or fairly prolonged period of time but then I would fall back into the regular routine. So, at the end in this 1960 I just made up my mind very determinedly that this thing wasn't going to beat me, I was going to beat it because it was ruining my relationship with my family. And sooner or later it was going to have an effect on my work. It hadn't up until then, fortunately, it never – it was never brought to my attention where I worked but it had a profound effect with my family.'

In cognitive social psychology, the Elaboration Likelihood Model [49] hypothesizes that attitude change will be more likely to occur and that a changed attitude will be more resistant to change if people are made to personally and deeply process the information on which the change will be based. Ideally people will come to formulate arguments in favor of the changed position. This reasoning process facilitates a linkage among thoughts supporting the change. Presumably such a linkage is one of the effects of a Decisional Balance exercise.

The experimental intervention in the FSC project was a motivational intervention where, based on the answers from their assessment materials, respondents were sent personalized feedback and a decisional balance exercise, all intended to enhance their motivation to change [4]. While the control group completed the same questionnaires as those in the experimental group, no personalized feedback was provided until their 12-month follow-up interview was completed. Similar to studies in the smoking field [63–66], respondents in the control group were given two informational pamphlets that provided information about the nature of alcohol abuse and general advice on how people could deal with their alcohol problem.

The one-year follow-up of the project has just been completed and the evaluation phase of the study is expected to be highly informative in terms of whether the personalized advice/feedback is successful in encouraging self-change and whether respondents who did not change sought other treatment.

EMPOWERING AND INVOLVING THE CONSUMER

In recent years, the term 'empowerment' has become popular [61, 67–69]. The term refers to individuals gaining control over their own lives, taking action on their own, and relying less on others for help. Dickerson [61] has asserted:

'Empowerment is an ideology that has emerged in reaction to inadequacies in systems of care for persons with serious mental illness' (p. 255).

In discussing the drug education strategies that embody zero-tolerance, scare tactics, no-use messages such as 'Just Say No,' and top-down teaching (i.e. don't involve teenagers, they have nothing to offer), Rosenbaum [67] says that such messages and programs not only fail, but also, by cutting off dialogue with young people, build resentment. When teenagers recognize they are being told what to do rather than being trusted to make informed decisions, they feel betrayed and angry. As an alternative, Rosenbaum [67] argues for a new drug education strategy that 'requires a pragmatic view that accepts the ability of teenagers, if educated honestly and in ways they trust, to make wise decisions, if not to abstinence, to moderate, controlled, and safe use' (p. 167).

In summary, according to Sobell [69] 'There is emerging evidence that empowering patients and addressing their psychosocial needs can be health and cost effective' (p. 237). Although empowerment is a new area of discussion and study, Dickerson [61] has identified different strategies and programs that might possibly foster empowerment, such as the 'clubhouse model of rehabilitation, self-help groups, consumers who work as providers, participatory action research, and advocacy activities'(p. 255). She also suggests that, while our traditional treatment may enhance a client's empowerment, to accomplish this 'Clinicians need to be sensitive to issues of stigma and disenfranchisement and to the social context of consumers' lives' (p. 255). Lastly, motivational interventions may foster that empowerment by recognizing and emphasizing people's strengths and resources [1]. Finally, in terms of dissemination research, our treatments and intervention and messages might be better received, accepted, and effective, if we involve consumers (i.e. those with problems) in services planning and delivery [70–72].

CONCLUSION AND FUTURE DIRECTIONS

Prevention and early intervention strategies are needed that are perceived as attractive and are sought rather than avoided. Despite the considerable cost to society of substance use and related problems, many individuals whose substance use might place them at risk have not experienced any consequences and do not consider their use as a problem.

The Fostering Self-Change intervention described in this chapter was designed to appeal to such individuals. This intervention is consistent with an efficient approach to public health care, in which individuals are first provided with an intervention that is least intrusive on their lifestyle yet has a reasonable chance of success [10, 11]. This and similar approaches have the opportunity of reaching large numbers of individuals who are otherwise unwilling, not ready, or not motivated to access the formal health care system. If such interventions succeed, it is reasonable to speculate that the change in respondents' behavior will have occurred earlier than would otherwise be expected and, therefore, that the anticipated costs to society of these respondents' substance use problems will be reduced. If the initial intervention does not work, the level of care can be stepped up (i.e. more treatment or an alternative treatment). Moreover, if these community interventions are successful they could then be employed and evaluated in a number of other settings (e.g. health care clinics, high schools and colleges, military bases).

REFERENCES

1. Substance Abuse and Mental Health Administration. Enhancing motivation for change in substance abuse treatment (Treatment Improvement Protocol Series No. 35). U.S. Department of Health and Human Services; Rockville, MD.
2. Miller, W.R. and Rollnick, S. (1991) *Motivational Interviewing: Preparing People to Change Addictive Behavior*, Guilford: New York.
3. Bandura, A. (1986) *Social Foundations of Thought and Action: A Social Cognitive Theory*, Prentice-Hall: Englewood Cliffs, NJ.
4. Sobell, L.C., Cunningham, J. and Sobell, M.B. *et al.* (1996) Fostering self-change among problem drinkers: A proactive community intervention. *Addict Behav.* 21(6), 817–833.
5. Fleming, M. and Manwell, L.B. (1999) Brief intervention in primary care settings: A primary treatment method for at-risk, problem, and dependent drinkers. *Alcohol Health Res World* 23(2), 128–137.
6. Heather, N. (1994) Brief interventions on the world map. *Addiction* **89**, 665–667.
7. Heather, N., Rollnick. S., Bell, A. and Richmond, R. (1996) Effects of brief counselling among male heavy drinkers identified on general hospital wards. *Drug Alcohol Rev.* 15(1), 29–38.
8. Sitharthan, T., Kavanagh, D.J. and Sayer, G. (1996) Moderating drinking by correspondence: An evaluation of a new method of intervention. *Addiction* 91(3), 345–355.
9. Sobell, M.B. and Sobell, L.C. (1993) *Problem Drinkers: Guided Self-change Treatment*, Guilford Press: New York.
10. Sobell, M.B. and Sobell, L.C. (1999) Stepped care for alcohol problems: An efficient method for planning and delivering clinical services, in *Changing Addictive Behavior: Bridging Clinical and Public Health Strategies* (eds J.A. Tucker, D.A. Donovan and G.A. Marlatt GA), Guilford Press: New York, pp. 331–343.
11. Sobell, M.B. and Sobell, L.C. (2000) Stepped care as a heuristic approach to the treatment of alcohol problems. *J Consult Clin Psychol.* **68**, 573–579.
12. Bien, T.H., Miller, W.R. and Tonigan, J.S. (1993) Brief interventions for alcohol problems: A review. *Addiction* **88**, 315–336.
13. Miller, W.R., Brown, J.M., Simpson, T.L. *et al.* (1995) What works? A methodological analysis of the alcohol treatment outcome literature, in *Handbook of Alcoholism Treatment Approaches: Effective Alternatives*, 2nd edn. (R.K. Hester and W.R. Miller), Allyn and Bacon: Boston, pp. 12–44.
14. Project MATCH Research Group. (1998) Matching alcoholism treatments to client heterogeneity: Project MATCH three-year drinking outcomes. *Alcohol: Clin Experiment Res.* **22**, 1300–1311.

15. Project MATCH Research Group. (1998) Matching alcoholism treatments to client heterogeneity: Treatment main effects and matching effects on drinking during treatment. *J Stud Alcohol* **59**(6), 631–639.
16. Sobell, M.B., Breslin, F.C. and Sobell, L.C. (1998) Project MATCH: The time has come ... to talk of many things. *J Stud Alcohol* **59**(1), 124–125.
17. Mahoney, M.J. and Lyddon, W.J. (1988) Recent developments in cognitive approaches to counseling and psychotherapy. *Counsel Psychol.* **16**, 190–234.
18. Thoresen, C.E. and Mahoney, M.J. (1974) *Behavioral Self-Control*, Rinehart and Winston: New York.
19. Sobell, M.B. and Sobell, L.C. (1998) Guiding self-change, in *Treating Addictive Behaviors*, 2nd edn (eds W.R. Miller and N. Heather), Plenum: New York, pp. 189–202.
20. Werch, C.E. (1990) Are drinkers interested in inexpensive approaches to reduce their alcohol use. *J Drug Educ.* **20**, 67–75.
21. National Institute on Alcohol Abuse and Alcoholism. (1995) The physicians' guide to helping patients with alcohol problems. National Institute on Alcohol Abuse and Alcoholism: Rockville, MD.
22. Breslin, C., Sobell, L.C., Sobell, M.B., Buchan, G. and Kwan, E. (1996) Aftercare telephone contacts with problem drinkers can serve a clinical and research function. *Addiction* **91**, 1359–1364.
23. Jeffery, R.W., Hellerstedt, W.L. and Schmid, T.L. (1990) Correspondence programs for smoking cessation and weight control: A comparison of two strategies in the Minnesota Heart Health Program. *Health Psychol.* **9**, 585–598.
24. Lando, H.A., Rolnick, S., Klevan, D., Roski, J., Cherney, L. and Lauger, G. (1997) Telephone support as an adjunct to transdermal nicotine in smoking cessation. *Am J Public Health* **87**(10), 1670–1674.
25. Ramelson, H.Z., Friedman, R.H. and Ockene, J.K. (1999) An automated telephone-based smoking cessation education and counseling system. *Patient Educ Couns.* **36**(2), 131–144.
26. Zhu, S.H., Stretch, V., Balabanis, M., Rosbrook, B., Sadler, G. and Pierce, J.P. (1996) Telephone counseling for smoking cessation: Effects of single-session and multiple-session interventions. *J Consult Clin Psychol.* **64**(1), 202–211.
27. Campion, P., Owen, L., Mcneill, A. and Mcguire, C. (1994) Evaluation of a mass media campaign on smoking and pregnancy. *Addiction* **89**, 1245–1254.
28. Giffen, C.A. (1991) Community intervention trial for smoking cessation (commit) – summary of design and intervention. *J Natl Cancer Inst.* **83**, 1620–1628.
29. Hughes, J.R., Cummings, K.M. and Hyland, A. (1999) Ability of smokers to reduce their smoking and its association with future smoking cessation. *Addiction* **94**(1), 109–114.
30. Killen, J.D., Fortmann, S.P., Newman, B. and Varady, A. (1990) Evaluation of a treatment approach combining nicotine gum with self-guided behavioral treatments for smoking relapse prevention. *J Consult Clin Psychol.* **58**, 85–92.
31. Lichtenstein, E., Lando, H.A. and Nothwehr, F. (1994) Readiness to quit as a predictor of smoking changes in the Minnesota Heart Health Program. *Health Psychol.* **13**, 393–396.
32. Pirie, P.L., Rooney, B.L., Pechacek, T.F., Lando, H.A. and Schmid, L.A. (1997) Incorporating social support into a community-wide smoking cessation contest. *Addict Behav.* **2**, 131–137.
33. Utz, S.W., Shuster, G.F., Merwin, E. and Williams, B. (1994) A community-based smoking-cessation program: Self-care behaviors and success. *Public Health Nurs.* **11**(5), 291–299.
34. Warner, K.E. (1981) Cigarette smoking in the 1970's: The impact of the antismoking campaign on consumption. *Science* **211**, 729–730.

35. Warner, K.E. (1989) Effects of the antismoking campaign: An update. *Am J Public Health* **79**, 144–151.
36. Alemi, F., Mosavel, M., Stephens, R.C., Ghadiri, A., Krishnaswamy, J. and Thakkar, H. (1996) Electronic self-help and support groups. *Med Care* **34**(10 Suppl.), OS32–OS44.
37. Wright, B., Williams, C. and Partridge, I. (1999) Management advice for children with chronic fatigue syndrome: a systematic study of information from the internet. *Irish J Psychol Med.* **16**(2), 67–71.
38. Heather, N. (1989) Psychology and brief interventions. *Br J Addict.* **84**, 357–370.
39. Sobell, L.C. and Sobell, M.B. (1992) Stability of natural recoveries from alcohol problems, in *Paper Presented at the Second International Conference on Behavioural Medicine*, 1992 July, Hamburg, Germany.
40. Sobell, L.C., Sobell, M.B., Toneatto, T. and Leo, G.I. (1993) What triggers the resolution of alcohol problems without treatment? *Alcohol: Clin Exp Res.* **17**(2), 217–224.
41. Chiauzzi, E.J. and Liljegren, S. (1993) Taboo topics in addiction treatment: An empirical review of clinical folklore. *J Subst Abuse Treat.* **10**, 303–316.
42. Cunningham, J.A., Sobell, L.C. and Chow, V.M.C. (1993) What's in a label? The effects of substance types and labels on treatment considerations and stigma. *J Stud Alcohol* **54**, 693–699.
43. Cunningham, J.A., Sobell, L.C., Sobell, M.B., Agrawal, S. and Toneatto, T. (1993) Barriers to treatment: Why alcohol and drug abusers delay or never seek treatment. *Addict Behav.* **18**, 347–353.
44. Grant, B.F. (1997) Barriers to alcoholism treatment: Reasons for not seeking treatment in a general population sample. *J Stud Alcohol* **58**(4), 365–371.
45. Klingemann, H.K.-H. (1991) The motivation for change from problem alcohol and heroin use. *Br J Addict.* **86**, 727–744.
46. Miller, W.R. and Hester, R.K. (1980) Treating the problem drinker: Modern approaches, in *The Addictive Behaviors: Treatment of Alcoholism, Drug Abuse, Smoking and Obesity* (ed. W.R. Miller), Pergamon Press: New York, pp. 11–141.
47. Miller, W.R., Taylor, C.A. and West, J.C. (1980) Focused versus broadspectrum behavior therapy for problem drinkers. *J Consult Clin Psychol.* **48**, 590–601.
48. Pearlman, S., Zweben, A. and Li, S. (1989) The comparability of solicited versus clinic subjects in alcohol treatment research. *Br J Addict.* **84**, 523–532.
49. Perloff, R.M. (1993) *The Dynamics of Persuasion*, Lawrence Erlbaum: Hillsdale, NJ.
50. Nadeau, L. (1997) The promotion of low-risk drinking styles: Sensitizing the public. A critical overview, in *Paper Presented at the Symposium on 'The Promotion of Low-Risk Drinking Patterns in the General Public: Strategies and Messages'*, 1997 October, Zurich, Switzerland.
51. Rehm, J. (1997) Campaigns and core messages: An up-to-date and state of the art from a research perspective? in *Paper Presented at the Symposium on 'The Promotion of Low-Risk Drinking Patterns in the General Public: Strategies and Messages'*, 1997 October, Zurich, Switzerland.
52. Hanna, E.Z., Chou, S.P. and Grant, B.F. (1997) Relationship between drinking and heart disease morbidity in the United States: Results from the National Health Interview Survey. *Alcohol: Clin Exp Res.* **21**, 111–118.
53. Svärdsudd, K. (1998) Moderate alcohol consumption and cardiovascular disease: Is there evidence for a preventive effect? *Alcohol: Clin Exp Res.* **22**(7), 307S–314S.
54. Dijkstra, A., DeVries, H., Roijackers, J. and vanBreukelen, G. (1998) Tailoring information to enhance quitting in smokers with low motivation to quit: Three basic efficacy questions. *Health Psychol.* **17**(6), 513–519.

55. Kreuter, M.W. and Strecher, V.J. (1996) Do tailored behavior change messages enhance the effectiveness of health risk appraisal? Results from a randomized trial. *Health Educ Res.* **11**, 97–105.
56. Skinner, C.S., Strecher, V.J. and Hospers, H. (1994) Physicians' recommendations for mammography: Do tailored messages make a difference? *Am J Public Health* **84**, 43–49.
57. Cunningham, J.A. (1999) Resolving alcohol-related problems with and without treatment: The effects of different problem criteria. *J Stud Alcohol* **60**(4), 463–466.
58. Sobell, L.C., Cunningham, J.A. and Sobell, M.B. (1996) Recovery from alcohol problems with and without treatment: Prevalence in two population surveys. *Am J Public Health* **86**(7), 966–972.
59. Cunningham, J.A., Sobell, L.C. and Freedman, J.L. (1994) Beliefs about the cause of substance abuse: A comparison of three drugs. *J Subst Abuse* **6**, 219–226.
60. Rush, B. and Allen, B.A. (1997) Attitudes and beliefs of the general public about treatment for alcohol problems. *Can J Public Health* **88**, 41–43.
61. Dickerson, F.B. (1998) Strategies that foster empowerment. *Cognitive and Behavioral Practice* **5**(2), 255–275.
62. Hingson, R., Mangione, T., Meyers, A. and Scotch, N. (1982) Seeking help for drinking problems: A study in the Boston metropolitan area. *J Stud Alcohol* **43**, 273–288.
63. Curry, S.J., McBride, C., Grothaus, L.C., Louie, D. and Wagner, E.H. (1995) A randomized trial of self-help materials, personalized feedback, and telephone counseling with nonvolunteer smokers. *J Consult Clin Psychol.* **63**, 1005–1014.
64. Dijkstra, A., DeVries, H., Roijackers, J. and vanBreukelen, G. (1998) Tailored interventions to communicate stage-matched information to smokers in different motivational stages. *J Consult Clin Psychol.* **66**, 549–557.
65. Ledwith, F. (1984) Immediate and delayed effects of postal advice on stopping smoking. *Health Bull.* **42**, 332–345.
66. Utz, S.W., Shuster, G.F., Merwin, E. and Williams, B. (1994) A community-based smoking-cessation program: Self-care behaviors and success. *Public Health Nurs.* **11**, 291–299.
67. Rosenbaum, M. (1998) 'Just say know' to teenagers and marijuana. *J Psychoactive Drugs* **30**(2), 197–203.
68. Rosenbaum, M. and Ronen, T. (1998) Clinical supervision from the standpoint of cognitive-behavior therapy. *Psychotherapy* **35**(2), 220–230.
69. Sobel, D.S. (1995) Rethinking medicine: Improving health outcomes with cost-effective psychosocial interventions. *Psychosom Med.* **57**(3), 234–244.
71. Martin, G.W., Herie, M.A., Turner, B.J. and Cunningham, J.A. (1998) A social marketing model for disseminating research-based treatments to addictions treatment providers. *Addiction* **93**(11), 1703–1715.
72. Rogers, E.M. (1995) *Diffusion of Innovations*, 4th edn, Free Press: New York.
73. Sobell, L.C. (1996) Bridging the gap between scientists and practitioners: The challenge before us. *Behav Ther.* **27**(3), 297–320.

Chapter nine

Environmental influences in natural resolution: bringing in context

Addiction perspectives on substance misuse focus on the allegedly irresistible appeal of alcohol or drugs among predisposed individuals, who presumably are made vulnerable to their addicting effects by some genetic, biological, or character flaw. An important shortcoming of this conventional perspective is that it ignores the powerful effects of the environmental context on alcohol and drug use, which is amenable to manipulation to reduce use and promote problem resolution. Ironically, interest in the environmental context that surrounds resolution of substance abuse problems has emerged from studies of natural recovery.

Research on natural recovery has highlighted the importance of social context, and of the resources that adhere to a person's social position, in the experience of self-resolution of addictive behavior [1–4]. In a recent paper, Blomqvist [5] argues that 'the way in which resources and life opportunities are allocated in the population are likely to influence peoples' overall options for stable recovery as well as the specific paths this process may take'. Similarly, Murphy and Rosenbaum [6] note that while virtually anyone can experience problems with alcohol and drugs, 'individuals with life options or [who] have a stake in conventional life tend to have a greater capacity for controlling their drug use or for getting out of trouble if they don't'.

While the social context that coheres to an individual's position within society has been viewed as relevant in natural recovery from addiction, a macro-level perspective that considers the importance of contextualized attributes on individuals, as well as of ecological characteristics present or absent within a community, remains under-theorized and under-researched. This chapter expands the theoretical discussions of natural recovery from addiction through an examination of the broader environmental factors that play a role in the self-resolution of alcohol and drug problems. This chapter begins with a discussion of a theoretical framework that operationalizes the environmental context of

> ### Resolved Alcohol Abuser
>
> 'And you know, the only time, since then, that I had a hard time was when I put myself in a situation. Stupid, absolutely stupid. I think it was that winter. It was that January, the following January. January '81, we went over to (name deleted) family. Just to spend a little time with them. I guess we went for Christmas, didn't we? '81? Or maybe it was in January or something. Anyway we were staying with her sister in a little town outside of (place) and we went out for dinner. And they were all drinking these glasses of wine and I knew exactly what it would taste like and I just knew it. I could smell it. I put myself in a dumb position. I really felt like I was being attacked by the enemy. He was saying, 'go on it will never hurt, never hurt.' I never had a desire to drink anymore, even then I didn't have a desire to drink, but I felt uncomfortable. Remember that? And then I just ordered an apple juice, I think, or malt. They have that malt, 'alcohol free malt drink', they call it and I had that. But it passed very quickly. But I realized that I put myself in the situation – I had done it.'

self-change. The social science concept of *social capital* is employed as a way of contextualizing substance abuse and its resolution. The concept of social capital is attractive because it provides a conceptual link between attributes of individuals and their immediate social contexts such as relationships and available community resources [7]. Next, we illustrate the value of this concept by exploring how preferences for substance use change as a function of environmentally based individual attributes as well as changing environmental circumstances. The chapter concludes with a discussion of the implications that our theorizing about natural recovery has for social policy, particularly for policies that complement a harm reduction perspective.

SOCIAL CAPITAL THEORY

Social scientists have increasingly used the term 'social capital' as a way of denoting the various types of resources appropriable from the interpersonal relationships within which a person is embedded [8]. Social capital is, as Bourdieu [9] postulates: 'the sum of the resources, actual or virtual, that accrue to an individual or a group by virtue of possessing a durable network of more or less institutionalized relationships of mutual acquaintance and recognition'. According to Coleman [10], social capital possesses a productive quality in its capacity to further self-interested pursuits. As he writes, social capital possesses:

. . . a variety of different entities having two characteristics in common: They all consist of some aspect of a social structure, and they facilitate certain action of individuals within the structure. Like other forms of capital, social capital is productive, making possible the achievement of certain ends that would not be attainable in its absence.

The resources that adhere to social relations can operate at the broader levels of social organization, as in the formation of civic groups and business norms pertaining to trust and cooperation, or they can adhere more locally to individuals within particular social settings [11, 12]. Embedded within individual's potential stock of social capital are the possibilities that they will benefit from their social relations.

Social capital can facilitate information diffusion, can restrict unfettered autonomy by creating normative expectations for reciprocity, and can provide

---

Recovered Heroin Addict

'The bad thing is the psyche, but because my friend stopped using heroin, I could do it too. Without that I would not have managed, I mean with people around me taking heroin I would not have mustered the force; after all it has been a quest for love and understanding and a place where I am accepted with all my weaknesses and faults.'

---

viable sources of social solidarity [8]. By investing in and accumulating capital that is based upon social relationships and community services, an individual potentially gains access to a wider array of resources that can be appropriated to motivate personal change that leads to improvements in life functioning.

For instance, individuals can utilize the personal networks and 'weak ties' of friends to acquire desirable jobs [13].

Also they can directly benefit from their parents' social capital expressed through community contacts, residential stability, high expectations, invest-

---

Recovered Cocaine Addict

'I came back and I made a phone call to a friend and I had a job. It was a good feeling, being able to do that after all I had been through, knowing that I can still get a job.'

---

ment of time, and social support, all of which leads to a greater tendency towards conventional behavior [14].

Access to social capital can lead to opportunities to become involved in community activities and services, develop commitments to pro-social activities,

---

Recovered Heroin Addict

'I [went] to a secluded house in the mountains owned by my dad . . . We [my husband and I] did it but I was miserable but I wasn't using. I think we were there for about 45 days.'

---

and establish healthy support systems necessary for wellbeing.

Thus, the amount and type of social capital that individuals are able to accumulate within the context in which they are embedded has significant

---

Recovered Alcohol Abuser

'I joined the Junior League . . . I signed up to be on [a] committee and ended up chairing it . . . I really have good female friends.'

---

implications for personal wellbeing and opportunities.

While the concept of social capital has been used to explain occupational mobility [13, 15] and civic culture [11] as well as business transactions, economic behavior and economic development more generally [10, 12, 16], it has utility also for understanding resolution of personal problems. Like the above examples, personal troubles such as substance abuse and its resolution are embedded within a larger structure of social relations and networks from which helpful resources may be obtained. Just as drug use is mediated by the structured relations within which one is embedded, so too are the opportunities for personal change.

As Murphy and Rosenbaum [6] assert, the opportunities for self-change among crack users in inner-city barrios are undoubtedly different from those in the middle class, who not only have better access to treatment but also possess greater amounts of social capital that can facilitate change. Indeed, higher status confers more resources, access to social relations, greater opportunities for self-change and, ultimately, enhanced quantities of social capital [17].

Recovered Alcohol Abuser

'Well I made up my mind. I was going to quit. I don't know how else I can explain it to you. It sounds simple I suppose to people who haven't been through it but the day, that evening rather, I went to the doctor and he gave me this good news and if it wasn't for my wife I wouldn't have thought about it, so when he told me, to this day I don't know whether it was true or not but I suspect it was, he knew our family. We all had a tendency to so when he told me what the alcohol was doing to my liver then I quit. I just went home and drank as much as I could as long as I could and whatever was left over the next morning went down the sink.'

APPLICATION TO HEALTH BEHAVIOR

Application of social capital theory to behavior associated with general health and wellbeing has emerged in recent years. For instance, Kawachi and his associates [18] cite data indicating a strong relationship between social capital and mortality rates within the general population. Research evidence presented by them supports the conclusion that social capital variables are related to differences in health outcomes. They found that communities with lower amounts of social capital generally had higher proportions of residents who reported having poor or only fair health. They asserted that social capital might influence health behavior in three distinct ways. First, social capital promotes a more rapid diffusion of health information, thereby increasing the likelihood that healthy norms of behavior are adopted, as well as increasing the likelihood of neighbors exerting some control over another's deviant behavior [18]. The amount of collective efficacy within a community, as measured by the extent a community is organized and is socially cohesive, leads to improvements in the general health of a community. Second, these authors suggested that neighborhood social capital may influence health by increasing access to local services and amenities such as community health clinics, recreational facilities, and educational facilities, which are all directly relevant to health. Indeed, research on natural recovery indicates that participation in alternatives to intoxicant use that are made available through social capital is critical to self-resolution of substance abuse [2, 19]. Finally, Kawachi and his associates [18, p. 1193] suggested that 'social capital may influence the health of individuals through psychosocial processes, by providing affective support and acting as the source of self-esteem and mutual respect'.

From this perspective, the broader networks and environments within which individuals are embedded significantly affect their levels of stress, self-efficacy,

---

Recovered Crack Addict

'When I stopped using crack and became affiliated with the Unitarian Church, I started to have some self-esteem and began to feel good about myself.'

Recovered Alcohol Abuser

'My kids and health . . . I want to be back in control of my health and my life again.'

---

and depression, all which are related to various types of ill health, including substance misuse.

A similar analysis by Hagan and McCarthy [20] has highlighted the critical importance of social capital in the lives of homeless young people. These authors found that their sample of homeless and criminal youth came from families with diminished social capital. These families neither offered social support to their children nor were able to connect their children to a stable aggregation of individuals or institutions in their neighborhoods. As these authors pointed out, social capital 'originates in socially structured relations between individuals, in families and in aggregations of individuals in neighborhoods' [20]. Additionally, since social capital adheres to communities as well as to individuals, these authors found that youth crime was differentiated across distinct community settings. Communities that provided few resources for alternative activities or invested little in social support services for youth tended to experience higher rates of youth crime. These youth were more likely to be in possession of criminal capital stemming from their embeddedness within street life. Lacking the social capital that flows from being embedded in conventional networks, such as employment, school and intact families, and in pro-social peer groups makes it increasingly more likely that these disadvantaged youth will engage in such behavior as delinquency, substance abuse, and dropping out of school [21–23].

By paying close attention to the embeddedness of behavior, the concept of social capital offers considerable utility for understanding problems associated with substance misuse and, particularly, their resolution without treatment. Individuals who overcome their alcohol and drug problems do so within a context of improved life circumstances and social relations. Self-remitters have been found to have reinvested in institutional life (i.e. family, work, education, religion, etc.) as well as to have developed or re-established meaningful social relationships, often within the social institutions to which they had been connected [2].

Recovered Alcohol Abuser

'I would say, I don't know if it's so much reinvent, but I changed, I think a great deal following the election and one of the ways that I changed was not drinking. And I, for me, it never was a task to quit drinking and to not drink. Or not a very difficult one at all, so I really didn't make an effort, that wasn't really my purpose. My purpose wasn't to quit drinking. My purpose was other things, to gain more self control and to be in control of myself, and one of the ways to go about that was to not drink.'

However, while these emerging institutional commitments and social relations proved beneficial to these self-remitters, they do not occur independent of each individual's embeddedness within a structured set of relations. In other words, people's ability to become immersed in conventional life, develop meaningful social relations and establish positive health habits is influenced by the social capital that exists prior to their substance misuse, by the amount of social capital they are able to retain while misusing drugs, and by the social capital that is available to them through their immediate communities.

Recovered Alcohol Abuser

'We lived in an affluent community. Our parents were members of the country club ... Then in college, in the fraternity, alcohol was plentiful and encouraged.'

The quality and quantity of social capital that drug and alcohol abusers possess assist them significantly in their level of motivation and attempts to improve their lives. Natural recovery from addictive behavior occurs in large part because of the particular structured social context of social relations within which substance misuse is embedded. The social capital that adheres to these relations can provide self-remitters with a variety of positive attributes, such as access to information, normative expectations, relationships, institutions, and other resources for their personal transformations, which might not otherwise be available in different social contexts [2].

Focusing on the broader contexts of substance misuse and behavior change offers the potential for significant insights, but it is a perspective that is underdeveloped and under-researched. Because the concept of social capital places emphasis on the capacity of people to solve their problems and improve their lives jointly with others [16], it can serve as a heuristic device for further understanding self-resolution of addictive problems, including the role of the surrounding environment in promoting positive change. In the next section, research findings on the environmental contexts that surround resolution of substance abuse are described.

These contexts include (1) the broader economic factors associated with drug use and cessation, (2) the availability of community services, and (3) improvements in individual life circumstances. As this section illustrates, policies that emphasize increasing the price and reducing the availability of drugs, which have dominated environmental approaches to the reduction of drug problems, are limited in scope. It is argued, however, that this is an unnecessarily narrow view of the role of the environment. It is suggested that an expanded perspective that also includes a focus on increasing social support services and non-drug alternatives within the community, as well as on enhancing personal networks and relationships, may help improve life functioning. The latter attributes, which are consistent with building social capital, deserve serious attention, in addition to the influential economic variables emphasized in research to date.

ECONOMIC INFLUENCES ON DRUG USE AND CESSATION OF USE

A substantial body of research, which is detailed in several recent books [24–26], has shown that drug use varies directly with the price of drugs and other constraints on drug access, and varies inversely with the availability of valued alternative activities that do not involve drug use. The main findings are summarized below. They indicate environmental features that increase the risk of substance use and abuse and, conversely, suggest ways that environments can be configured to reduce drug use and related problems.

- Price affects demand for licit and illicit drugs, as measured by the number of users, quantities consumed, and indices of drug-related harm [25]. As the full price of drugs increases, demand decreases, and vice versa. Thus, drugs function as a 'normal good' in that demand for them is governed by the basic law of supply and demand. This general relation holds across a wide range of substances and user groups and indicates that demand can be reduced by raising the full price of drugs.

- Drug use by youths is especially sensitive to price changes, more so than among adults, especially those with established drug-taking habits. Raising drug prices, therefore, helps decrease or delay the acquisition of drug use (e.g. smoking, alcohol use) among adolescents and young adults [25].

- Other interventions that constrain drug availability, such as restricting the hours of operation of bars and liquor outlets or limiting smoking in worksite and public locations, can reduce drug use [27].

- The effectiveness of interventions aimed at constraining drug use and making drugs more expensive depends critically on what other activities and commodities are available. If the broader environment is bereft of alternative non-drug reinforcers that can compete with drug use, drug preferences will remain high, and further increases in drug prices will promote the development of a black market and increase criminal activity associated with drug-seeking behavior [28]. Moreover, income and drug use tend to be inversely related, and decreases in income reduce non-drug consumption to a greater degree than drug use [29].

- Conversely, enriching the broader environment with attractive non-drug alternatives, including opportunities for employment and social interaction, reduces the demand for drugs, even if the price of drugs is relatively low. Environmental enrichment also retards the initial acquisition of drug use, which has important implications for effective prevention programming for youths [29, 30].

Overall, these findings indicate that substance use and the harm it causes can be reduced by the implementation of policies that increase drug prices, decrease drug availability, and increase the availability of valued alternative activities. However, policies that only emphasize increasing the price and reducing the availability of drugs often create new problems, such as increasing drug-related crime and discouraging the use of helping resources by persons with problems [31]. The US War on Drugs epitomizes this approach and its associated problems.

EXPANDING HELPING RESOURCES FOR SUBSTANCE ABUSERS

The interventions available to persons in need are another environmental feature that influences the likelihood and ease of change in addictive behavior. Until recently, intensive specialized treatments, which best serve the needs of the minority of persons with more serious problems, were the dominant form of professional help available. Such treatments are 'high threshold', stigmatizing, and typically require abstinence for entry and continued participation [32]. Most persons affected find them unappealing and prefer to attempt to resolve their problems on their own, with the aid of family and friends, or by participation in mutual help groups. Although help from informal sources works for some, and others recover without identifiable assistance from any source, there has been a conspicuous gap in professional helping resources for individuals who do not require intensive treatment but who could benefit from some assistance beyond that offered by the voluntary sector. Moreover, intensive treatment slots are not evenly distributed and do not meet the needs of significant segments of the drug-abusing community. In the United States, for example, slots in private treatment programs go unused, while addicts wait for months for a place in publicly funded methadone treatment programs in urban areas.

Recovered Alcohol Abuser

'I can't afford to go into [hospitals]. Too expensive. There again no one can do it but yourself.'

Several European countries (e.g. the Netherlands, Switzerland) have made considerable progress in expanding services to better serve the diversity of problems associated with substance misuse [31]. Specialized formal treatment has been supplemented with briefer interventions offered in community, primary care, and other non-traditional settings. These interventions are important for several reasons:

- They facilitate naturally occurring changes that may lead to problem resolution without subjecting individuals with less serious problems to interventions that are unnecessarily costly, disruptive, and sweeping in scope [33].

- They reduce the harm or risk of harm associated with substance use, even if abstinence is not attainable; e.g. clean needle exchanges reduce the spread of HIV among injection drug users, their sex partners, and offspring [34].

- They increase access to services and create a continuum of care that matches the continuum of substance-related problems [35].

- They serve as low-threshold pathways for onward referrals to needed medical care or specialized substance abuse treatment [36, 37].

- They are consumer-oriented and address problems of living associated with addictive behavior, which is a primary motive for help-seeking, and they do not restrict their focus to eliminating substance use [32].

Thus, expanding the range and goals of services and making them more accessible are important environmental considerations in an overall strategy to reduce substance misuse and the problems it causes. As stated by Tapert and colleagues [38], the goal should be: 'Make it as easy to get services as it is to get drugs' (p. 183).

INDIVIDUAL LIFE CONTEXTS SURROUNDING NATURAL RESOLUTION

In addition to broad environmental features such as the economic context of drug-taking and the availability of alternative non-drug reinforcers and helping resources, there are environmental variables that operate on a more individual level to affect the likelihood of change in addictive behavior, including natural resolution. Although the elimination of abusive substance use by individuals is often a fairly time-limited event with an identifiable onset, this discrete act typically is surrounded in time by reliable changes in individuals' life circumstances, which appear to motivate and maintain positive change. Over a period of several years surrounding initial change, successful long-term resolutions are associated with increases in negative events prior to initial change. These negative events typically occur in areas of functioning that are adversely affected by addictive behavior (e.g. family and social relations; health, work, and legal problems) and appear to help motivate resolution attempts.

Recovered Cocaine Addict

'My performance [at work] went downhill, which meant the income went downhill, so less money. I wasn't going to slack up on the coke so I slacked up on the bills.'

Recovered Alcohol Abuser

'I've seen the positive effect of where my business is going and where I am putting my money. Growing up – putting my money into tangible things. Decided that's what I wanted, was a reason not to drink.'

Following initial behavior change, increases in positive events and improvements in life functioning (e.g. in social relations, positive health habits) are common in successful resolutions, especially during the first year of maintenance, and appear to reinforce continued maintenance efforts. This general pattern has been observed in studies of natural resolution from alcohol [4, 39, 40], drugs [5, 41], gambling [42], obesity [43], and eating [44] disorders. Of the two sets of event patterns, the improved life contexts that occur during maintenance have been more consistently observed, particularly in prospective research [4, 39].

This work indicates that resolution often is a lengthy process that unfolds over several years, even though the act of initiating abstinence or moderating addictive behavior patterns may be fairly discrete. The maintenance interval appears to be a key phase in the resolution process; it merits greater investigation and more attention in intervention programs, which typically focus on initiating change, more than on maintaining it.

Recovered Alcohol Abuser through Treatment and AA

'I look for ways to divert myself and my attitudes away from drinking towards other activities that would keep me engrossed enough to keep from drinking.'

Recovered Alcohol Abuser

'[I] exercise more, eat better, [am] teaching myself to feel good.'

Although commonalities exist across addictive behavior in the general contexts that are associated with natural resolutions, differences have been observed that are disorder-specific. For example, compared with problem drinkers who resolve their problems, abusers of such illicit drugs as opiates and amphetamines tend to be more marginalized and to have experienced more drug-related difficulties. Thus, they usually have to make more pervasive changes in their life context in order to resolve their problem [5]. As another example, positive financial changes appear to be more influential in helping maintain gambling resolution than substance abuse resolution [42].

Another key issue is the extent to which a core set of environmental variables is associated with resolution achieved with and without interventions and what unique contributions interventions make in promoting change, as well as when this typically occurs. Preliminary research suggests that both assisted and natural resolution is supported by similar environmental contexts that reflect improvements across the pre-resolution through the post-resolution intervals [4, 5, 40, 44]. In addition to these shared contextual characteristics, interventions, especially formal treatment, have been found to enhance the positive changes that occur during maintenance, especially during the first year after initial change. Furthermore, many individuals who seek help tend to do so after they have made some initial changes on their own, including the initiation of abstinence in the case of substance abuse [5, 45]. These findings further emphasize the probable importance of improved life circumstances during maintenance in supporting stable behavior change, suggest that interventions may facilitate such changes, and indicate that some affected individuals enter interventions in order to consolidate behavior changes that they had already initiated themselves.

FUTURE DIRECTIONS

The environmental conditions supporting self-resolution from substance misuse have numerous implications for treatment and policy initiatives. As this chapter has pointed out, self-change from addictive behavior occurs in a broader context of networks, resources, community investments, and overall improvements in life circumstances within which an individual is embedded. It is this *embedded* quality of self-resolution that makes an emphasis on broader environmental contexts important to consider. Overall, the critical insight offered by bringing context into an understanding of self-change is the importance of building an individual's capacity to engage in a process of self-change [17, 31]. As suggested by this chapter, the environmental conditions and social capital within which an individual is embedded can serve to enhance the individual's capacity to overcome substance misuse problems without treatment.

Enhancing capacity to overcome alcohol, drug, and nicotine problems is an intervention that is consistent with general principles of harm reduction. At its most basic level, harm reduction connotes individual and group efforts to optimize the health of drug users in order to reduce secondary harm associated with use. Needle exchange, tolerance zones, and safe-injection rooms are common types of harm reduction efforts. This chapter suggests that harm reduction efforts should move beyond these traditional approaches to address the broader context of use and misuse [31]. In addition to direct initiatives and interventions, harm reduction work should also move toward exploring ways in which the broader environments can be shaped to enhance the capacity to overcome substance related problems. It is in this area that harm reduction advocates could find utility in the concept of social capital. As Erikson [46] suggests, 'the building of social capital to bring about the improvement of the most fundamental living conditions of the population is a vital aspect of harm reduction'. Investigations that focus on enhancing the capacity for self-resolution through improvements in social capital may be a fruitful research agenda for the future.

REFERENCES

1. Granfield, R. and Cloud, W. (1996) The elephant that no one sees: Natural recovery among middle-class addicts. *J Drug Iss.* **26**(1), 45–61.
2. Granfield, R. and Cloud, W. (1999) *Coming Clean: Overcoming Addiction Without Treatment*, New York University Press: New York.
3. Tucker, J.A., Vuchinich, R.E. and Gladsjo, J.A. (1990) Environmental events surrounding natural recovery from alcohol-related problems. *J Stud Alcohol* **25**, 1017–1050.
4. Tucker, J.A. (1999) Environmental contexts surrounding resolution among problem drinkers with different help-seeking experiences. Paper presented at *Thematic Meeting on the Natural History of Addictions Hosted by the Swiss Institute for the Prevention of Alcohol and other Drug Problems*, Les Diablerets, Switzerland.

5.   Blomqvist, J. (1999) Recovery with and without treatment: A comparison of resolutions of alcohol and drug problems. Paper presented at *Thematic Meeting on the Natural History of Addictions Hosted by the Swiss Institute for the Prevention of Alcohol and other Drug Problems*, Les Diablerets, Switzerland.
6.   Murphy, S. and Rosenbaum, M. (1997) Two women who used cocaine too much: Class, race, gender, crack and coke, in *Crack in Context: Demon Drugs and Social Justice* (eds C. Reinarman and H.G. Levine), University of California Press: Berkeley, CA.
7.   Furstenberg, F. and Hughes, M. (1995) Social capital and successful development among at-risk youth. *J Marriage Fam.* **57**, 580–592.
8.   Sandefur, R. and Laumann, E. (1998) A paradigm for social capital. *Rationality Soc.* **10**, 481–501.
9.   Bourdieu, P. and Wacquant, J.D. (1992) *An Invitation to Reflexive Sociology*, University of Chicago Press: Chicago.
10. Coleman, J. (1990) *Foundation of Social Theory*, Harvard University Press: Cambridge, Massachusetts.
11. Putnam, R. (1993) *Making Democracy Work: Civic Tradition in Modern Italy*, Princeton University Press: Princeton, New Jersey.
12. Fukuyama, F. (1995) *Trust: The Social Virtues and The Creation of Prosperity*, Free Press: New York.
13. Granovetter, M. (1974) *Getting a Job: A Study of Contacts and Careers*, Harvard University Press: Cambridge, Massachusetts.
14. Runyan, D., Hunter, W., Socolar, R.S. and Amaya-Jackson, R.L. (1998) Children who prosper in unfavorable environments: The relationship to social capital. *Pediatrics*, **10**, 12–18.
15. Granfield, R. and Koenig, T. (1992) Pathways to elite law firms: Professional stratification and social networks, in *Research on Politics and Society* (eds G. Moore and A. Whitt), JAI Press: Greenwich, Connecticut.
16. Flora, J. (1998) Social capital and communities of place. *Rural Sociol.* **63**, 481–506.
17. Kiecolt, J. (1994) Stress and the decision to change oneself: A theoretical model. *Soc Psychol Q.* **57**, 49–63.
18. Kawachi, I.B., Kennedy, B. and Glass, R. (1999) Social capital and self-rated health: A contextual analysis. *Am J Public Health* **98**, 1187–1193.
19. Biernacki, P. (1986) *Pathways from Heroin Addiction: Recovery without Treatment*, Temple University Press: Philadelphia.
20. Hagan, J. and McCarthy, B. (1997) *Mean Streets: Youth, Crime and Homelessness*, Cambridge University Press: Cambridge, UK.
21. Teachman, J., Paasch, K. and Carver, K. Social capital and the generation of human capital. *Soc Forces* **74**(4), 1343–1359.
22. Sullivan, M. (1990) *Getting Paid: Youth Crime and Work in the Inner City*, Cornell University Press: Ithica.
23. Hawkins, J.D., Catelano, R.F. and Miller, J.Y. (1992) Risk and protective factors for alcohol and other drug problems in adolescence and early adulthood: Implications for substance abuse prevention. *Psychol Bull.* **112**, 64–105.
24. Bickel, W.K. and Vuchinich, R.E. (eds) (2000) *Reframing Health Behavior Change with Behavioral Economics*, Lawrence Erlbaum Associates: Mahwah, NJ.
25. Chaloupka, F.J., Grossman, M., Bickel, W.K. and Saffer, H. (eds) (1999) *The Economic Analysis of Substance Use and Abuse: An Integration of Economic and Behavioral Economic Research*, University of Chicago Press: Chicago, IL.
26. Green, L. and Kagel, J.H. (eds) (1996) *Advances in Behavioral Economics*, Ablex Publishing Co.: Norwood, NJ.
27. Ohsfeldt, R.L., Boyle, R.G. and Capilouto, E.I. (1999) Tobacco taxes, smoking restrictions, and tobacco use, in *The Economic Analysis of Substance Use and Abuse:*

An Integration of Econometric and Behavioral Economic Research (eds F.J. Chaloupka, M. Grossman, W.K. Bickel and H. Saffer), University of Chicago Press: Chicago, IL, pp. 15–30.

28. Bickel, W.R. and DeGrandpre, R.J. (1995) Price and alternatives: Suggestions for drug policy from psychology. *Int J Drug Policy* **6**, 93–105.

29. Carroll, M.E. (1999) Income alters the relative reinforcing effects of drug and nondrug reinforcers, in *The Economic Analysis of Substance Use and Abuse: An Integration of Econometric and Behavioral Economic Research* (eds F.J. Chaloupka, M. Grossman, W.K. Bickel and H. Saffer), University of Chicago Press: Chicago, IL, pp. 311–326.

30. Fisher, E.B. (1996) A behavioral-economic perspective on the influence of social support on cigarette smoking, in *Advances in Behavioral Economics* (eds L. Green and J.H. Kagel), Ablex Publishing Co.: Norwood, NJ.

31. Marlatt, G.A. (1998) *Harm Reduction: Pragmatic Strategies for Managing High-Risk Behaviors*, Guilford Press: New York.

32. Marlatt, G.A., Tucker, J.A., Donovan, D.A. and Vuchinich, R.E. (1997) Help-seeking by substance abusers: The role of harm reduction and the role of behavioral-economic approaches to facilitate treatment entry and retention, in *Beyond the Therapeutic Alliance: Keeping the Drug-Dependent Individual in Treatment* (eds L.S. Onken, J.D. Blaine and J.J. Boren) (Research Monograph No 165). Rockville, MD: National Institute of Drug Abuse, pp. 44–84.

33. Tucker, J.A. (1999) Changing addictive behavior: Historical and contemporary perspectives, in *Changing Addictive Behavior: Bridging Clinical and Public Health Strategies* (eds J.A. Tucker, D.A. Donovan and G.A. Marlatt), Guilford Press: New York, pp. 3–44.

34. U.S. National Institute of Health. (1997) Interventions to prevent HIV risk behaviors, Bethesda, MD.

35. Institute of Medicine. (1990) *Broadening the Base of Treatment for Alcohol Problems*, National Academy Press: Washington, DC.

36. Zweben, A. and Fleming, M.F. (1999) Brief interventions for alcohol and drug problems, in *Changing Addictive Behavior: Bridging Clinical and Public Health Strategies* (eds J.A. Tucker, D.A. Donovan and G.A. Marlatt), Guilford Press: New York, pp. 251–282.

37. Carvell, A.M. and Hart, G.J. (1990) Help-seeking and referrals in a needle exchange: A comprehensive service to injecting drug users. *Br J Addict.* **85**, 235–240.

38. Tapert, S.F., Kilmer, J.R., Quiqley, L.A., Larimer, M.E., Roberts, L.J. and Miller, E.T. (1998) Harm reduction strategies for illicit substance use and abuse, in *Harm Reduction: Pragmatic Strategies for Managing High Risk Behaviors* (ed. G.A. Marlatt), Guilford Press: New York, pp. 145–217.

39. Humphreys, K., Moos, R.H. and Finney, J.W. (1995) Two pathways out of drinking problems without professional treatment. *Addict Behav.* **20**(4), 427–441.

40. Tucker, J.A., Vuchinich, R.E. and Pukish, M.M. (1995) Molar environmental contexts surrounding recovery by treated and untreated problem drinkers. *Exp Clin Psychopharmacol.* **3**, 195–204.

41. Klingemann, H.K.-H. (1991) The motivation for change from problem alcohol and heroin use. *Br J Addict.* **86**, 727–744.

42. Hodgins, D.C. (1999) Natural and treatment-assisted recovery from gambling problems: a comparison of resolved and active gamblers. Paper presented at *International Conference on Natural History of Addictions: Recovery from Alcohol, Tobacco, and Other Drug Problems Without Treatment*, March 7–12, 1999, Les Diablerets, Switzerland.

43. Tinker, J.E. and Tucker, J.A. (1997) Environmental events surrounding natural recovery from obesity. *Addict Behav.* **22**, 571–575.
44. Crawford, A.L. and Tucker, J.A. (2000) Life events surrounding behavior change efforts and treatment entry among women with bulimia nervosa (unpublished manuscript).
45. Tucker, J.A. (1995) Predictors of help-seeking and the temporal relationship of help to recovery among treated and untreated recovered problem drinkers. *Addiction* **90**(6), 805–809.
46. Erikson, P. (1999) Harm reduction among cocaine users: Reflexions on individual intervention and community social capital. *Int J Drug Policy* **10**, 235–246.

Chapter ten

Natural recovery in cross-cultural perspective

As we have already seen, the idea of 'natural recovery' or 'spontaneous remission' from various states of addiction is a poorly understood and much contested concept. Some commentators in the field of alcohol and drug studies accept that it happens, while others remain skeptical. Given the nature of this debate occurring within Anglo-European societies, it is not surprising to find that the idea of natural recovery becomes even more problematic and unclear when considering other non-Western societies. Regrettably, little cross-cultural research has been done on these issues, so we lack specific knowledge. Indeed, Klingemann [1, p. 155] notes the dominance of the USA in the literature – of 80 works reviewed on environmental influences impeding or promoting change in substance behavior by adolescents, seven came from outside the US and only one from a non-anglophone country.

In this chapter, then, we use information about alcohol and drug use and abuse from a broad range of cultural settings to bring relevant questions to the fore. We do this to sensitize therapists and interested others to the range and depth of issues underlying work with addicted individuals from different cultural backgrounds. Such attention to cross-cultural issues is important. First, it allows practitioners dealing with refugee or migrant populations from non-Western nations to understand how they might differ from dominant Anglo-European populations in attitude or response to problem substance use or addiction [2]. Second, such a focus allows a more refined understanding of underlying concepts and assumptions central to promoting self-change or 'natural recovery' from problem substance use, i.e. concepts and issues such as 'disease', 'addiction', 'treatment', 'drug abuse', 'dependency' and 'control'.

CROSS-CULTURAL VARIATION IN BELIEFS AND NORMATIVE BEHAVIOR

Underlying the ideas of 'recovery' and 'treatment' are notions of disease or unacceptably disordered behavior versus well-being or normatively proper behavior. Such notions intrinsically influence opportunities and means for self-change or natural recovery. Ideas such as these vary widely, not just by culture, but also by historical era, population demographics, prevailing theories of medicine, the degree of socially approved latitude in behavior, and modes of social control [3]. For example, it is common for highland Peruvian peasants to chew coca leaves and ingest the juice as a necessary adjunct or stimulant to work, whereas in the West cocaine, the refined substance extracted from coca leaves, has no generally accepted image as a beneficial substance. In early 19th century Europe, absinthe was a fashionable drink among the urban middle class until it was banned some decades later because of its deleterious – even deadly – effects on physical well-being and social life. Cigarette smoking by adults, especially males, is tolerated in most societies, whereas frequently smoking by children or females is heavily punished [4, 5]. Whether excessive consumption of alcohol is a disease/addiction or a symptom/result of a disordered life has been hotly debated in the literature; whether moderate consumption of alcohol leads to physical health benefits is equally contested. What comprises 'excessive' or 'moderate' consumption is equally disputed. In many non-Western societies, alcohol abuse, even when it results in domestic violence or public displays of lewd or enraged behavior, is viewed as a regrettable but intrinsic characteristic of an individual for which he or she is not responsible, a characteristic made visible, but not caused by drinking.

Among Cook Islanders in the Pacific, a drunken brawl is not just a mechanism for release of aggression, but also a culturally approved means to point up and punish in public infractions of family and community morals [6, p. 48]. Strict distinctions may be drawn by gender; for example, drunkenness by women, whether due to ingestion of alcohol or of kava, a local brew from *Piper methysticum*, is not tolerated in most Western Pacific societies [7]. Chewing of betel (*Areca catechu*) is a widespread custom throughout Asia and the Pacific, yet this stimulant is barely recognized in the West, nor is there much research on its pharmacological properties, let alone its social uses [7].

What is normal, natural and proper in one society seems strange, disturbing, and repulsive in another. Understood in context, however, each society's assumptions and behavior become comprehensible and rational. For example, in certain South American Indian groups, male shamans (specialist healers and seers) deliberately ingest hallucinogens in order to invoke communication with the gods, especially about important and socially central activities such as warfare or hunting expeditions. Moreover, they will often blow the same substances into the nostrils of their hunting dogs to enhance the animals' abilities to detect game so essential to survival. In contrast, most Western cultures view very negatively any but the most mildly altered state of consciousness or cognitive ability, any loss of control, especially when these states are induced deliberately or chemically. Pharmacologically-active substances, however, such as alcohol, kava, betel, tobacco, ginger, mushrooms and other fungi, the bark of various trees, and exudates from insects, amphibians or plants, are all widely used to stimulate altered physiological or cognitive states, to induce or enhance out-of-body or out-of-mind experiences. The boundary between food, medicine, cosmetic, religious material and drug is blurred, particularly outside American or European settings [8, 9].

CULTURAL TYPES: BROADLY DRAWN

No social or cultural group is homogeneous. Within every group, some people know more about, or are more interested in, health issues than are other people. Often these people are recognized within their society as health professionals – shamans, acupuncturists, chiropractors, homeopathic practitioners, midwives, dentists or surgeons – with an elaborated medical knowledge and recognized set of beliefs and practices. Generally, people are pragmatic about treatment, seeking and using anything that provides relief, and people will change behavior around illness far more readily than they will change their underlying beliefs about the cause of the disorder. The more similar a patient and healer, in age, sex, ethnicity, religion, education, occupational status, geographic location (e.g. rural vs. urban setting) and socio-economic class, the more likely they are to hold the same health beliefs and to engage in mutually comprehensible behavior [2, 3].

Health beliefs alone do not explain why people act, react or think in the way they do. Basic cultural values and assumptions about the nature of life; proper ways of relating to various categories of people, animals and objects; and behavioral norms and expectations – in short, worldview or general orientation to life – all help form a people's health beliefs or explanatory models [10].

Recovered Alcohol Abuser

'Being a nice person, being in control, being healthy, being intelligent. Those all good things. I guess those are all values, like you said earlier, and those are things that I strive for. That I work towards. And it's one, it's not greater than anything else. Being healthy is not greater than being intelligent or being in control, but they're several aspects of the right, the good kind of person.'

To understand how worldview can affect therapeutic endeavors, we present here two different cultural styles [11, 12]. These represent extremes, and our presentation deliberately highlights the differences so that the impact of these orientations becomes clear [13]. Most cultural groups, however, hold more nuanced, less strident, more middle-of-the-range views that nevertheless draw on, and are informed by, the ideas presented here.

Specialist cultures

The first cultural style is the Western, or Anglo-European. This culture has been characterized as 'specialist' in orientation [11–13]. Basic mottoes of life in specialist cultures seem to be: 'Every person for himself or herself' and 'Keep your eye on the prize.' Specialist cultures are future oriented, actively seeking to prevent problems. Time is a commodity that can be spent, wasted, donated or saved. Specialist cultures are also technologically innovative, deliberately seeking to devise and use new therapies and healing devices. They are egalitarian, secular, and heavily focussed on the individual and independence. A model of the proper-life course is a 'shooting star' – a steep, straight upward trajectory ending in a blaze of glory. In other words, through education and accumulation of personal wealth, anyone can and should achieve, should rise rapidly in individual esteem, renown, capability, and wealth, i.e. should quickly fulfill their potential. Specialist cultures prize health, for educational and financial successes depend on it. They tend to distinguish physical from mental/emotional health. Physical health is 'correctable' through appropriate diagnosis and treatment with medications or surgery, whereas mental or emotional disorders are seen as fundamentally disruptive of the social fabric and result in marginalization of the sufferer. In such an individualistic society, one has to have a strong and stable sense of self that is able to act independently in and on the world because no one else can help one achieve life's goals. Addiction to alcohol or drugs is extremely disruptive to achievement of an individual's ability to reach full potential.

Anglo-European cultures represent variations on this idea of specialist culture. Despite being so fundamentally similar, they can differ markedly in their attitudes towards use and abuse of alcohol and drugs. So-called 'wet' cultures, such as France and Spain, are liberal in permitting access to alcohol, and tolerant in their treatment of problems arising from abuse. In contrast, Scandinavian countries, so-called 'dry' cultures, strictly control access to addictive substances such as alcohol and tend to be more punitive in their responses to alcohol and drug abuse [14, 15]. Moreover, the premium choice of alcoholic beverage varies widely between Southern and Northern European countries – wine (fermented) vs. vodka (distilled) – a difference due partly to agriculture, economics and trade, partly to historical precedent, and partly to complex cultural symbolism and ideology. Intra-national differences can be as profound as inter-national ones; e.g. the drinking rate for the German-speaking cultural population in Switzerland has decreased since 1981, unlike the alcohol consumption rate for the general Swiss population, which has remained steady [1, p. 150]. Just as differences within specialist cultures can sometimes be crucial in terms of attitude and practice, so can they be relatively mute. Sobell and colleagues [16], for example, found that people in Switzerland and Canada used very similar processes of cognitive evaluation and assessment to spur natural remission from alcohol and drug abuse.

Generalist cultures

In contrast to Anglo-European cultures, many non-Western cultures can be described as 'generalist' cultures, with an 'up-n-down, roller coaster' model of the individual life course [11–13]. Such cultures are portrayed as present-oriented and motivated more by immediate need to accomplish a task than by future planning or prevention of problems. These are hierarchical, sacred/religious, traditional cultures with a strong focus on family and group interconnections or interdependence. Fundamental guiding mottoes seem to be: 'Go with the flow' and 'Enjoy the ride.' Individual achievement, through education or wealth accumulation, is good as long as the outcomes can and are redistributed to benefit everyone in the family. Health is valued but sometimes an individual has to forgo or wait for treatment if some other family member's need is more urgent. Illness is often accepted with a degree of stoicism or fatalism, and mental and physical health is often not separated. A person suffering from mental and emotional distress remains a valued member able to contribute something, however meager, to the family. To survive in a group with this basic life trajectory, one needs a mobile, flexible sense of self that is able to adapt to various contingencies and to sublimate individual desire for collective good. Time is not a commodity so much as a flexible medium in which one lives in the here-and-now, and so one does not worry about things over which one has no control, such as the future. Indeed, individual ability to control life is not a major concern and is often deliberately eschewed in order to achieve other culturally desirable ends. In these societies, an addicted individual would be less disruptive of familial or community life [17].

As among specialist cultures, there is variation among and within generalist cultures in attitude and practice in connection with alcohol, drugs, and other substances or addictive habits. This is well documented in the comparative literature on alcohol and drug treatment. The Latin-influenced nations of Peru and Colombia, for example, deal with drug addiction largely through voluntary treatment in non-governmental organizations whereas the East Asian nations of China and Japan resort to compulsory detoxification in formal government controlled units [14, 15].

Ethnic minorities and mainstream populations

'How I started with my drinking was with the European, when I was only young then I get involved with European ways of living. In that time I got deeper and deeper involved in alcoholism. At the end I was stupid, I didn't know what was going on I was blindfold by the alcoholic spirit. Its poison to us, mainly. The Aboriginal people because we can't handle it, because it's not our culture in other words.' [18, p. 96]

Today it is common to find populations from generalist cultures within main-stream Anglo-European specialist cultures. Over the past two decades there has been massive migration of non-Western peoples into European countries (e.g. Turks in Germany, Indonesians in Holland, Algerians in France, West Africans and West Indians in Britain), into various Anglo-affiliated countries (e.g. East Indians in Canada, Pacific Islanders in New Zealand and Australia), and into the United States (e.g. Asians, Latinos, Afghanis, Ethiopians, Haitians). These migrant groups bring attitudes, knowledge and use practices with respect to alcohol and drugs that vary from the mainstream Anglo-European populations. Such differences often but not always become muted over time, with second or third generation ethnic minorities approaching the mainstream pattern of consumption and beliefs. For example, Kitano and colleagues [19, 20] report that Japanese men in Japan were far less accepting of drinking by women, and were heavier consumers of alcohol, than Japanese-American men born and raised in Hawaii. Religious Jews, however, tend to be abstemious consumers of alcohol, no matter where in the world they live or how long they have been there.

'Well, at the time, when I got a taste of it I thought it was good for me, I didn't know, I was blindfold – no-one ever taught Aboriginal people all the wide world, no-one ever taught us what alcohol could do to our people. We just got in, just like cattle in a trough, just like Jack and few other people saying, we just go straight into the trough and have as much as we can drink.' [18, p. 97]

Despite the presence of multiple, distinct, non-Western or other generalist populations in most major Anglo-European cities worldwide, there is little literature on normative practices of substance use or abuse by these minority or ethnic groups. Stereotypes about such groups often substitute for careful research-based knowledge, and unresolved conceptual issues abound. These shortcomings not only are under-acknowledged by researchers and clinicians, but also seriously diminish the utility of the existing literature. We consider here in some detail the case of Asian Americans, not because they are unique or special in the degree to which they represent conceptual and methodological problems, but rather because they illustrate so well issues common to under-standing minority/ethnic populations everywhere. People at present fleeing into various European nations are Croatian or Serbian, Muslim or Christian, wealthy or poor, from rural and urban areas. As long as researchers, clinicians, social welfare workers, and government agents identify them simply as 'refugees from Kosovo', knowledge about their attitudes towards, and use of, addictive substances will be no more adequate than the information about Asian Americans.

Asian Americans

The United States Census Bureau officially aggregates all people of Asian origin into a single category: 'Asian Pacific Islander,' a term encompassing at least 60 distinct, named ethnic groups from more than 20 different nations [21]. Some of these Asian ethnic groups (e.g. Chinese and Japanese) have been in the USA since the 1850s and have large, generationally complex, well-established communities in metropolitan areas. Other Asian groups have been in the USA for only two decades (e.g. Cambodians or Laotians, recent refugees from South-East Asia) and comprise smaller, economically struggling enclaves of shallow generational depth. National origin is often used as a descriptor – e.g. Chinese, Vietnamese, Guamanian. While more fine-grained than the census term, the national-origin term does not eliminate problems arising from important social, cultural, historical and linguistic differences. The Hmong and the Iu-Mien, for example, are two distinct ethnic groups from the highlands of South-East Asia, a region overlapping the national borders of Laos, Cambodia, Vietnam, and Thailand. Until 30 years ago, opium was a major cash crop in this region, especially for the Iu-Mien, and older members of these groups often still regard this drug as a useful home remedy for many everyday maladies. Further, 'Vietnamese' as a descriptor makes no distinction between a person with origins in a Vietnamese cultural group and a person with origins in a migrant, ethnic Chinese group resident in Vietnam. While 'China' might be an unambiguous descriptor of geographic or national origin, it makes no allowance for differences due to language or dialect (e.g. Cantonese vs. Mandarin). Nor does it indicate whether a person comes from the dominant Han ethnic group or from the Dai or the Hakka, to name but a few of the more than 30 minority ethnic groups in China. Recording and reporting the specific name of the ethnic group as recognized and used by its members, as well as their nation of origin, would go a long way towards overcoming some inadequacies in available data.

For many years, a common stereotype of Asians in the US has been that they constitute a 'model minority' – a quiet, law-abiding, hard-working, family-oriented group that excels educationally and is economically successful [22]. When data about Asians in the US are disaggregated, however, a severe challenge is issued to this stereotype. Instead of 'model minority', a more complex picture emerges, of different histories, of a broad range of distinctive settlement and demographic patterns and of widespread variations in wealth, health and longevity [21, 23, 24]. Also evident are distinct patterns of practice and belief about substance use and abuse, especially around alcohol and smoking. For example, well-established Asian communities tend to have smoking rates similar to general US rates, between 25% and 30%, depending on sex and age. Newer Asian immigrant groups, such as those from Cambodia or

Vietnam, are distinctly different: Fewer women in these populations smoke (usually less than 20%, even as low as 5% for some age groups) but many more men smoke, over 50%, even as high as 65% for some age groups [25]. There is evidence, too, that alcohol and drug prevalence rates also vary by specific Asian ethnicity, as well as by age and sex [21, 26, 27].

The stereotype of 'model minority' has prevented social welfare and health officials from recognizing diversity within the Asian community and from dealing with both short- and long-term consequences of migration stress, especially among refugees. These under-recognized stresses are often due to role reversals: (a) between children and parents when it is only the children who speak English or understand the American way of life or bureaucratic system; and (b) between spouses, especially when it is only the wife who can obtain a job. Inter-generational tensions also exist, when grandparents are no longer accorded respect or obedience or can no longer communicate with their mono-lingual English-speaking grandchildren, or when children shed allegiance to animistic, Taoist, Confucian, Buddhist, Shinto, Hinduism or other non-Abraha-mic religions to adopt Christianity but their parents and grandparents do not. Life events, such as death of a parent or spouse, divorce, severe illness or trauma, or the up-rooting act of migration itself, have been associated with prompting or exacerbating substance use. Personal evaluation of the meaning of life events and role changes, and of their multiple long-term consequences, however, seems to have as much, if not greater, potential for negatively affecting self-esteem and for increasing substance use [1]. While the specific mechanisms remain unclear, the stresses and tensions outlined above have led some Asians, youth in particular, to increasingly poor educational performance, increasing alienation from family and community, increasing gang membership, increasing violence and criminal activity, and increasing substance use and abuse [22].

SOME CENTRAL DOMAINS FOR SELF-CHANGE

Cross-cultural differences with respect to addiction and recovery will be vividly displayed around five domains: namely, definition and trajectory of the problem behavior from onset to recovery, concepts and use of time, management and display of emotions and affect, sense of identity, and access and resort to experts. There is, of course, a great deal of overlap between these domains, which serves to reinforce the point that they comprise heuristic rather than intrinsic distinctions. This overlap also serves to reinforce the idea that addiction and recovery are complex notions, inextricably intertwined with cultural values, social behavior and environmental (treatment/recovery) contexts. Within each domain, we pose some central questions about its influence on the nature of self-improvement or spontaneous recovery, and provide a brief commentary and pertinent illustrations.

Problem definition and trajectory

- How, when and by whom do substances come to be classed as 'dangerous' or 'addictive'?

- What are the definition and progression of the illness or addicted state and the trajectory of recovery?

- How, when, and where can this trajectory be interrupted through spontaneous recovery or professional treatment?

- For or from what is recovery or treatment sought? What is being treated – behavior or patho-physiology?

- From addiction to, or abuse of, substances or from what non-normative behavior is recovery sought – excess alcohol consumption, food, illegal drugs, legal drugs, other types of addictive behavior?

- Who becomes addicted and who needs to recover?

'The publican asked me if I had a permit and I said 'what the hell's a permit?' and he said 'are you an Aboriginal?', I said 'yeah'. In no uncertain terms he called me a black so-and-so and to get out of there. So I hopped the bar and clobbered him and I was arrested and I said 'why are you arresting me, why don't you arrest the barman?' and they said 'because you're an Aboriginal'. I said 'what that's got to do with it?' and they said 'you're not allowed to drink alcohol.' ' [18, p. 162]

Definitions of substances as legal or illegal, beneficial or harmful, controlled or commercially available often produce the 'problem' being 'treated' and the need for 'recovery.' Moreover, there is wide variation in what different nations, populations or cultural groups deem to be a 'drug', not to mention differences between lay-public and professional definitions. For example, *khat* (variously known also as *qat, gat* or *chat*) is a plant-derived medicine/drug (*Catha edulis*) widely used by Somali, Yemeni or Ethiopian populations [28]. In Europe and North America, physicians or counselors unfamiliar with these migrant communities often have not heard of this plant, let alone know of its psychoactive properties. There could well be a sizeable proportion of people in such ethnic groups who resort to such drugs. Precisely because most research is focused so heavily on substances better known and more commonly used in Western societies, examining 'natural recovery' in these groups will almost certainly miss important cultural underpinnings unless the therapist is open to, and active in, discovering new information. Furthermore, recovery from addiction to such 'exotic' substances, if it occurs at all, may involve the input or intervention of other individuals in societies (healers from the local community, family members or even friends) in ways that are markedly different from those more familiar to mainstream professionals.

Even within dominant populations in Western societies, different groups vary in their categorizations of, and response to, addiction, be they government officials, healing practitioners, or ordinary citizens. Among professional treatment practitioners (e.g. physicians, social workers, counselors) concerned with managing or monitoring the effects of psychoactive substances, definitions of addiction change over time. For example, beneficial legal drugs are officially listed and controlled by legislation and prescription by certain licensed professionals. The addictive qualities of many of these drugs (e.g. Valium®) were not recognized initially, in part at least because it was mainly middle-class, white housewives in urban areas who were being prescribed them. Unlike other segments of the population (such as, ethnic minorities, adolescents, blue-collar workers), that particular demographic group is not usually viewed as having a drug problem, or constituting a 'dangerous class' in society [29]. Even when recognized, the addictive qualities did not force these therapeutic products from the market, in large part because these 'addicts' were not societally disruptive. Rather, it remains legal for a physician to prescribe such compounds without regulated follow-up or monitoring of outcome, though general awareness has been heightened about the potential for problem outcomes. With a few notable exceptions, ceasing to use these licit addictive substances/drugs is not categorized as 'recovery.' Currently, one might need to recover from using marijuana as a recreational pursuit in Anglo-European society, but would one need to recover if it were being used as a medicine, a re-classification that many groups of patients with specific conditions (e.g. glaucoma) would like to occur? Not all substances alleged (or known) to have psychoactive properties are yet officially recognized or regulated as drugs in Anglo-European countries. Some examples are herbal preparations, such as St. John's wort, or the class of compounds coming to be called *nutriceuticals* – 'foods' containing some substances, such as vitamins and minerals or similar products, alleged to have some vital pharmacological or therapeutic properties. Until recently, the possibility of addiction to, or need to recover from reliance on, these kinds of substances had not been raised.

Throughout the 20th century in Western societies tobacco was a legal substance fairly readily available to all adults. Moreover, it is a highly addictive substance from which the majority of former smokers 'recovered' spontaneously. Estimates suggest that as many as 70% or more former smokers quit without any form of professional help, other than public education campaigns [16]. Despite the enormous scale of this instance of natural recovery, we know extraordinarily little about it. These later examples highlight the sociopolitical-economic nature of many decisions concerning the classification of drugs and, hence, concerning the need for, or the possibility of, natural recovery from reliance or use.

Given these potential differences in problem definition, steps taken to 'cure' the malady will change from culture to culture. For example, the notion of addiction as a longlasting disease, especially one that cannot be cured but only held in remission, may not exist in non-Western societies.

An illness which persists is sometimes viewed as having been improperly cured, for once a good cure from a good healer is administered the illness will disappear. Alternatively, a persistent illness is sometimes said to have originated through sorcery, witchcraft, or evil directed towards the sufferer, the removal of which is necessary before cure can be successful [30].

Recovered Alcohol Abuser

'So the desire is gone and this is where I part company with Alcoholics Anonymous and people like them, because they operate on a naturalistic bias. A naturalistic way whereas not necessarily Alcoholics Anonymous, because AA started as a Christian organization. But they say you are always an alcoholic. And I say no I am no longer an alcoholic because I have been totally cured. And in second Corintheans, v.17, it says that if any man is in Christ, he is a new creation. All things have passed away before all things have become new. And I have just taken that verse, it may be out of context, but I have taken that verse as my particular inspiration that I am no longer an alcoholic.'

Time

- When in a person's life is addiction likely to occur and recovery generally expected to take place? (e.g. at what age or social stage, e.g. youth, marriage, birth of first child, or widowhood). In what life circumstances do specific 'triggers' for addiction or recovery operate (e.g. death of a parent, birth of a grandchild)?

- What is the trajectory or sequence of expected change(s) that mark recovery?

- What is the expected endpoint of recovery? Is recovery expected to be permanent and robust or a persistently fragile accomplishment?

- What temporal patterns in daily or ceremonial life facilitate or hinder recovery?

In every culture, one's occupation or productive economic/subsistence activity is probably the most important mechanism for structuring everyday life. Work permits the development of a regular temporal sequence of events and behavioral opportunities, (e.g. when to eat, sleep, take one's leisure, or participate in family or community ceremonies or rituals). These are reflected, too, in diurnal patterns of officially permitted access to legal substances, such as, the hours during which a pharmacy, pub, or liquor store is open. Temporal sequencing of daily life is highly diverse cross-culturally. To take just one small example, the number of meals per day, the times they are taken, when the main meal is consumed, how meals interface with other activities, all vary widely from group to group. Americans travelling in Italy, for example, are often startled to discover that many shops, schools and businesses close for two to three hours in the middle of the day so that everyone can go home to eat and have a nap. And these travellers are surprised to find that in the evening restaurants do not open for dinner until much later than is customary in the USA – often well after 7 pm, even as 'late' as 9 pm.

Hours for work or leisure vary not only by the nature of the job available but also by socially expected and approved patterns of interaction. Many refugees in Anglo-European cities work as janitors or watchmen, who usually work at night, and so have different rhythms for eating and sleeping, and thus different access to alcohol or cigarettes. In some Middle Eastern societies, for example, a man is expected to meet regularly at local coffee bars with kin, friends and clients to exchange news and gossip .

In Lebanon, consumption of *arak*, a powerful alcoholic aperitif, is an important social lubricant, often accompanying a lengthy meal during which men conduct business.

Brady [18] points to a seasonality in drunkenness among rural Australian Aborigines, noting weekday 'dry spells' versus weekend 'binges.' Seasonality is often evident in the consequences of drunkenness, too. In Papua New Guinea, for example, there are more fatal drunk-driving crashes at weekends than on weekdays [31]. How do family, friends, and professionals (be they licensed or local healing experts) assist in maintaining normative patterns of daily or seasonal behavior? When and how are addictive substances incorporated into the temporal sequences of life? How does work act to increase, reduce or ameliorate addictive behavior?

Addicts, especially those unable to maintain employment, find it extraordinarily difficult to uphold the structure of everyday life [17]. Indeed, their temporal sequencing often comes to revolve entirely around finding the next 'hit' or drink in order to stay high or inebriated. Further, their activities become increasingly clandestine, especially if addicted to an illegal substance. Recovery – or at least being on the way to recovery – is often indicated by once more engaging in the same temporal pattern of activities as the non-addicted. Professional programs aimed at assisting recovery can sometimes unwittingly be counterproductive. For example, methadone maintenance clinics in the USA frequently disrupt an addict's attempt to maintain full-time employment because they are open only during normal week-day working hours [32].

Sudden conversion experiences have been recorded, such as when a person renounces alcohol or finds God. Indeed, religious conversion was a major reason some Australian Aborigines cited for 'giving away the grog' [18].

Recovered Alcohol Abuser

'I was reading a Christian book, I was drinking a drink, I put it down on the counter, I went into my parents bedroom, they were not there, and I got on my knees ... And I admitted in prayer to the Lord the fact that I was an alcoholic and that I was now asking for his help to heal me and to cure me of alcoholism ... I prayed that would happen, and I thanked the Lord and I claimed it and I believed. And I got up, poured out the drink that I was drinking, and I never even finished it ... Got on the airplane because I knew from the minute that I got off my knees that I was healed.'

Complete cessation of problem consumption is the accepted endpoint in many Anglo-European settings; significant moderation of use of the addictive substance is an acceptable endpoint or state of recovery in many other cultures [15]. It might be easier to cut down to acceptable levels or to refrain from substance use entirely in a context where temporary abstinence from prized activity is culturally appropriate (e.g. during Lent for active Christians). In the Anglo-American world, however, total abstinence is frequently claimed to be the only acceptable state, the mark of complete recovery.

Emotion

- What is the range of emotions normally permitted for expression and what are the form and circumstances proper for doing so? By whom and when are particular kinds of emotional display improper?

- What affective states are permitted? Which of them make people uncomfortable?

- What is the role of social or community forces outside the individual (e.g. family, professionals in law and order, medicine, spirituality) in mediating and ameliorating troublesome behavior, especially that due to alcohol or drug use?

- How is display of emotion affected by addiction, and how is it supposed to change in recovery?

Most cultures generally do not approve the unfettered expression of all emotional states, but mask some states while allowing others free rein [33, 34]. In specialist, Anglo-European societies, for example, joy, pleasure, amusement, cheerfulness are states that are positively valued and can be overtly manifest in most circumstances without needing to be muted or explained. Sadness, puzzlement, shyness, irritation, distress, fright, worry, grief can also be expressed but not for too long or too forcefully, for these are less approved emotions. Strong negative emotions – anger, rage, terror – are rarely permitted, and are supposed to be quickly squelched. Thus, from a European drunkard, singing and loud maudlin sentimentality is more acceptable than vituperative rage or physically aggressive anger. Noisy, shambling drunken behavior may still make others uneasy or wary, but it is far more acceptable than bursts of profanity or violence.

Years ago, MacAndrew and Edgerton [35] coined the phrase 'drunken comportment' to describe how alcoholics learn to behave in a culturally approved fashion when inebriated. In Western societies, it is common for others to withdraw from the presence of drugged/drunken/enraged persons, to leave them 'to cool off' by themselves. Such a tactic acknowledges the centrality of the individual, his essential independence from others, and the need for him to regain control of himself by himself. Withdrawal does not work well in generalist cultures, where interdependence is key. For example, among Polynesians, it is important that trusted friends or family remain present to ameliorate and contain a person's (drunken) rage. This ensures that group norms of acceptable emotions and displays of behavior are modeled, and that the person is drawn back into the circle of relationships, not excluded from it. The drunk man is placated precisely because his rage is legitimated through public acknowledgement.

Different cultures have different standards for comportment when 'under the influence' of alcohol or drugs or in emotional pain. This is easily overlooked in the heat of the moment when police, social services or health care workers have to deal with drunk or drugged members of different cultural groups – or when it appears that someone is drunk. Consider Ethiopians, for example, a soft-spoken, mild-mannered people not given to loud or public displays of emotion. For them, however, the proper emotional and behavioral response on hearing of the death of a loved one is immediate, loud, uncontrolled wailing and screaming, the flailing of limbs, and the literal tearing of clothes and hair, especially as family and friends gather in response to the news [36]. Neighbors often seriously misinterpret such sudden, dramatic and unaccustomed changes in demeanor, ascribing these outbursts of 'wild' behavior to drunkenness or drug use and calling in the police to restore order. This has led to considerable misunder-standing and anger between civil authorities trying to 'keep the peace' and Ethiopians trying to mourn properly their loved one, especially when the behavior is accompanied by incompletely understood explanations in unfami-liar languages.

Western cultures are highly rationalist and focused on a rather concrete, empirical reality. Generally, in these cultures, people are very uneasy in the presence of those who hallucinate or have affective patterns different from the norm. Those who are actively dementing, delirious or hallucinating, whether for organic or for chemical reasons, make others nervous and uneasy and are therefore often shunned [3, 34]. Conversely, in many other cultures, talking to long dead ancestors, or seeing or hearing people, noises or activity not apparent to others, is not a suspect activity, even if stimulated by plant or chemical ingestion. Rather, hallucinatory or other altered sensory states are often highly regarded, as signs of an important ability to establish direct contact with spirits or a parallel world.

Identity

- Is the addicted person's 'deviant status' privately or publicly acknowledged?

- What is conceived to be the possibility of 'change' in identity – i.e. is a person seen as having a 'career' as a drug addict or alcoholic as, say, in the West, or as having a persona or personality characteristic as a bully or argumentative person, which is exacerbated by alcohol or drugs, as in many non-Western cultures ?

- How does the role of outside forces (e.g. family, healing expert) articulate with ideas of independence, control, and self/identity?

- What is the link between identity and social position (life trajectory/age/ chronology issues, especially developmental stage, gender differences, and within-group socio-economic class differences)?

- Who is thought to be 'at risk' for need of recovery, and how and when should they be treated (men, women, children, animals)?

The acceptability of non-normative behavior varies significantly by age, gender, ethnicity, socio-economic class, and geographic location. Thus, for example, among low-income adults over age 65 in rural settings in the United States, it is found that a much smaller proportion of women than of men smoke. Not only do such women smoke far fewer cigarettes than their male counterparts, but also they smoke less than women of younger age, or of the same age but with higher incomes or living in an urban location. Social expectations and rules around inappropriate behavior, both now and when these women were younger, helped shape this finding. When these women were young adults, smoking (especially in public) was not only a declaration of rebellion but also acceptance, albeit often reluctantly, of a reputation as 'easy' or 'loose' women. In general, far fewer older women than older men willingly quit smoking [37].

A major difference between Western/Anglo-European cultures and non-Western cultures is the degree to which stigmatization of the addicted person occurs, the degree to which the addict is viewed as deviant [5]. In Western cultures, whether deviancy be due to criminal activity (e.g. stealing to support a drug habit), personal inadequacy (e.g. drinking to excess), or functional rather than organic illness (e.g. mental or emotional conditions), extrusion of the deviant from family and from the wider society commonly occurs. Should remission from the problem take place, be it due to natural recovery or through professional therapeutic encounters, the person is re-integrated into main-stream society, though usually still with a 'suspect' label as a 'recovering' addict. Sometimes, the deviant label is so indelible, the extrusion so permanent, that people who share a particular outcast status band together to form sub-cultural groups, each with its own values and norms of behavior (e.g. the homeless mentally ill, or injection drug users).

Consistent with the values of generalist cultures, in non-Western settings mental or emotional illness or addiction frequently does not result in extreme social marginalization [5]. While the family or community may condemn the behavior, they rarely carry over that condemnation to include the actual person himself or herself. Rather, the individual remains within the family circle and receives public support for his or her efforts to deal with addiction. In some West African societies, for example, possession cults exist. These are organizations which sufferers join in order to express collectively through dance, trance and chant their mental or emotional anguish, and to display their affliction and non-normative behavior in a public place to a mainstream audience of non-members [33, 34]. Their addiction/illness is not shameful, nor is it kept secret. Compare this with a therapeutic self-help group in the West, such as Alcoholics Anonymous. Here meetings are held out of sight of the general public, and while each member is supported on an individual journey to recovery there is not the same kind of collective celebration or acceptance of the disease or addiction that unites group members.

Expertise

- Who properly can treat various states of altered consciousness?

- Does recovery involve 'experts' or not? If so, an expert in what?

- Does the 'recovered' person pay? Whom? How? What?

- Where does recovery take place (home vs. community setting vs. special other location)?

- What procedures or means are used to treat (e.g. fasting, sweat lodges, herbal medicines)? How could these be used to facilitate self-change or spontaneous remission?

Professionals can have a profound influence on an addict's desire and resolve to quit, depending on when in the addict's life this intervention comes. Health was the primary reason that Australian Aborigines gave for spontaneously quitting drinking, after some physician or nurse or other respected expert told them 'knock it off or die' [18].

> 'Then she took me up and I went in the hospital here. The doctor said 'you're sick from drinking too much'. And they had a plastic bag that shifted through my nose and a plastic bag down here and they drained it out, a bottle of moselle and beer, I think that what I was drinking. They flew me up in Darwin Hospital and I still had that tube and thing through my nose and I had that operation. My liver and kidney was really bad, and I was told from doctor not to be drinking anymore because I sick. You see, doctor told me, 'if you drink again you should have been dead.' ' [18 p. 32]

What this also means, however, is that the alcoholic or drug user has to have been consuming for a long enough period of time or heavily enough that some deleterious physical effect is evident, and that he or she has reached a life stage where no longer drinking, smoking, snorting, sniffing, or injecting is acceptable. A young adult, especially a male, in the prime of life may be teased or tormented by peers for not drinking alcohol, whereas an older adult may be excused. Both Australian Aborigines [18] and urban American Indians [38] comment on how drunkenness is actually unacceptable at older ages, especially as a person adopts, willingly or otherwise, certain central, highly valued social roles, such as becoming a grandparent. In other societies, a change in an important social role, such as getting married, has frequently been cited by former problem drinkers or drug users as a reason for spontaneously quitting [39].

If the client and the expert come from the same cultural backgrounds, it is likely that they will share the same cultural assumptions about both the origins of the addiction and the possible need for treatment. However, if client and treatment practitioner do not, there may be cultural misunderstandings. For example, in Western societies, the precise procedures adopted during treatment are generally perceived as a somewhat private affair, even if group methods are adopted; whereas in many non-Western societies treatment processes may be seen primarily as a social event, not solely for the purpose of the patient but also for the community – a process Kleinman [10] calls 'cultural healing.' In other words, in such societies the healing process acts as an integrative process restoring both group cohesion and individual integration. Once the client's disruptive behavior has been resolved, the healing process works to repay obligations incurred while the individual was ill.

Although developed within a specific cultural system, treatment modalities are often 'exported' or 'imported' across national boundaries, depending on the political and policy climate with respect to substance use and treatment [40, 41]. While Anglo-European countries frequently take the lead in devising and exporting/importing treatment methods (e.g. the Liverpool experiments in England, the Swiss heroin trials, and various 12-Step Programs from the United States), the development and export of treatment is not limited to Western settings – *naikan* therapy, for example, a group-oriented personal-insight therapeutic approach that originated in Japan, is now used in a number of other countries, including in Europe [42]. The success of exported treatment modalities is variable, especially among population groups for which the therapy was not originally designed [40].

The role the family is expected to play in treatment varies widely, even within European countries [41]. In Western societies discussing one's problems, either with friends or with professionals, may be viewed as a way of finding a solution to the problems, whereas keeping problems hidden is often seen as 'dangerous'. However, in other societies, openly discussing 'illnesses' or 'problems' outside the close-knit extended family group may be seen as dangerous, and the best way forward is to keep problems private. Reasons for this may involve politics and socio-economic status within the community, as well as stigma. Outside help can be an uncomfortable and public admission of family failure to cure or at least control the condition. Chin [43], for example, recounts how a migrant Korean family's attempts to manage at home a severely mentally ill son eventually fell apart, to their distress and shame. Where treatment is sought outside the family, it frequently involves trusted others with whom family members have long-standing complex relations, such as a business patron or a spiritual guide, such as a priest or shaman. Galanti [2] provides case examples of the many different types of relationship that can exist between patients and healers in non-Western cultural groups. Among migrant populations, these healers and group leaders can often be usefully incorporated into therapeutic situations involving members of their group.

Furthermore, if the individual's illness is perceived as the result of some malevolent behavior on the part of others in the community, part of the healing process may entail reparation from those who are suspected of causing the misfortune. Frequently reparation involves not just the afflicted transgressing individual but also his or her wider family or clan. Only after reparation has taken place can the community become integrated again. Joining with other family or community members to make reparation could be a major way in which 'spontaneous recovery' takes place. This process is fundamentally different to the process of healing in Western societies. There, once an individual has become labeled as an addict or drug dependant, he or she becomes separated or alienated from the rest of the society, even after treatment. Unlike other illnesses, the drug addict or the alcoholic remains in the state of being in recovery. Consequently, unlike many non-Western societies, the societal process of labeling erects barriers around individuals and separates them from the social groups of which they are part.

In examining the role of the expert in non-Western societies, the case of the shaman is particularly important. In nations with few trained professionals or accredited clinics for the treatment of problem substance use, indigenous healers, such as shamans, become key resources, as Lara-Ponce [44] has noted for rural Peru. In cases of possession, a state similar to that of the dependent substance user, to return the individual to a prior state the shaman may adopt practices whereby he allows himself to become possessed by the same spirits as those of the possessed person. However, as Lewis [45] notes, whereas the state of possession for the shaman is controlled, the possession for the client is not. In this state of 'controlled abnormality' the shaman is able to master or neutralize the spirits, those afflicting not just himself but also his clients [46]. Shamanic control occurs in two realms – that of symbolic ritual and that of physiological/psychological process. What comforts the mind and soul heals and cures the body.

CONCLUSION

This brief outline shows how the idea of 'spontaneous remission' or 'natural recovery' becomes exceptionally problematic but extremely instructive when considered cross-culturally. Therapists, counselors, and others working with people from minority cultures who are undergoing recovery from an addiction, need to be very aware of the impact of cross-cultural differences. They need to appreciate the crucial role played by the social location of the problem substance user, and of how social forces work in both the minority and the mainstream cultures.

Within all cultural groups, social location and social forces affect definitions, values, and behavior related to addictive substances, especially alcohol and drugs. The social location of the addict or person in recovery (i.e. age, gender, ethnicity, socio-economic class, and geographic and historical cohort) affects access to, and use of, particular substances. Wider social forces impinging on the individual (e.g. laws and regulations, resources such as treatment clinics or social services, social policies) directly impact an individual's access to, and success with, treatment. Practitioners need to be alert to cues that 'problems' with, and recovery from, alcohol and drug use may be manifest in quite distinct ways in different cultural groups.

While it is desirable that counselors and therapists not only speak the language of their minority clients but also are aware of key cultural values and behavioral norms, this is usually exceptionally difficult to achieve when dealing with multiple distinct minority groups. In the absence of such detailed knowledge, it is imperative that treatment professionals learn to recognize central issues around which many miscommunications occur [13]. These are most likely to be:

- Ideas about basic trajectory of life and its goals

- Range of allowable expression of emotions

- Time patterning of everyday behavior, especially work

- Beliefs and behavior in connection with addictive substances, the course of illnesses in general and substance abuse in particular, the trajectory of recovery and evidence for success in treatment

- Issues of identity, stigma, and independence

- Notions of family as a source of decision-making, as having authority over individual members, and as a care-giving unit. Awareness of generational differences, especially in migrant groups

- Resort to experts to assist in recovery.

Differences in the impact of social location and social forces become even more marked and complex when assisting a client from a minority group as opposed to a mainstream one. Such differences, especially between specialist (e.g. Western or Anglo-European) and generalist (e.g. non-Western) groups, carry important implications for the global 'export/import' of addiction treatments very broadly defined, including the concept of 'natural recovery' or 'spontaneous remission'. The more specific the information you know about your clients and their cultural affiliation, the more helpful it will be. Seek to know the name, the geographic origin and historical background of a minority group, as well as its demographic and health profile. Be wary of lumping into unitary categories groups that are distinct, and eschew stereotypes. Remember that difficulties and miscommunications are not caused by minority clients or by mainstream therapists but are, rather, the result of two different cultural systems in interaction. Whenever unexpected things happen or difficulties arise in treating a client from a different cultural group, consult an expert. The best expert is a bilingual, bi-cultural person knowledgeable about both minority and mainstream populations, a respected individual who through culturally appropriate and sensitive translation can help resolve the impasse stemming from different backgrounds, expectations, and experience.

REFERENCES

1. Klingemann, H.K.H. (1994) Environmental influences which promote or impede change in substance behaviour, in *Addiction: Processes of Change* (eds G. Edwards and M. Lader), Oxford University Press: Oxford, pp. 131–161.
2. Galanti, G.A. (1991) *Caring for Patients from Different Cultures*, University of Pennsylvania Press: Philadelphia.
3. Good, B. (1986) Explanatory models and care-seeking: A critical account, in *Illness Behavior: A Multidisciplinary Model* (eds S. McHugh and T.M. Vallis), Plenum: New York.

4. Gusfield, J.R. (1993) The social symbolism of smoking and health, in *Smoking Policy: Law, Politics and Culture* (eds S. Sugarman S and R. Rabin), Oxford University Press: New York.
5. Knipe, E. (1995) *Culture, Society and Drugs: The Social Science Approach to Drug Use*, Waveland Press: Prospect Heights, Ill.
6. Banwell, C. (1989) *The Place of Alcohol in the Lives of Cook Island Women Living in Auckland*, Department of Anthropology, University of Auckland: Auckland, Report no. 2.
7. Marshall, M. (1987) An overview of drugs in Oceania, in *Drugs in Western Pacific Societies: Relations of Substance* (ed. I. Lindstrom), University Press of America: New York.
8. Dobkin de Rios, M. (1984) *Hallucinogens: Cross-Cultural Perspectives*, University of New Mexico Press: Albuquerque.
9. Etkin, N.L. (1996) Ethnopharmacology, in *Medical Anthropology: Contemporary Theory and Methods*, revised edition (eds C.F. Sargent and T.M. Johnson), Praeger: Westport.
10. Kleinman, A. (1980) *Patients and Healers in the Context of Culture: An Exploration of the Borderland between Anthropology, Medicine and Psychiatry*, University of California Press: Berkeley.
11. Hall, E.T. (1956) *The Hidden Dimension*, Doubleday: Garden City, NY.
12. Hall, E.T. (1959) *The Silent Language*, Doubleday: Garden City, NY.
13. Barker, J.C. (1994) Recognizing cultural differences: Health-care providers and elderly patients. *Gerontol Geriatr Educ.* **15**, 9–21.
14. Klingemann, H. and Hunt, G. (1998) *Drug Treatment Systems in an International Perspective*, Sage Publications Inc.: Thousand Oaks, CA.
15. Klingemann, H., Takala, J.P. and Hunt, G. (1992) *Cure, Care, or Control: Alcoholism Treatment in Sixteen Countries*, State University of New York Press: Albany, NY.
16. Sobell, L.C., Klingemann, H., Toneatto, T., Sobell, M.B., Agrawal, S. and Leo, G.I. (unpublished manuscript) Computer-assisted content analysis of alcohol and drug abusers' perceived reasons for self-change in Canada and Switzerland.
17. Klingemann, H.K.H. (2000) 'To every thing there is a season' – social time and clock time in addiction treatment. *Soc Sci Med.* **5**, 99–108.
18. Brady, M. (1993) Giving away the grog: An ethnography of Aboriginal drinkers who quit without help. *Drug Alcohol Rev.* **12**, 401–411.
19. Kitano, H.H.I., Chi, I., Law, C.K., Lubben, J.E. and Rhee, S. (1988) Alcohol consumption of Japanese in Japan, Hawaii and California, in *Cultural Influences and Drinking Patterns* (eds L.H. Towle and T.C. Hartford), Government Printing Office: Washington DC.
20. Kitano, H.H.I., Chi, I., Rhee, S. and Lubben, J.E. (1992) Norms and alcohol consumption: Japanese in Japan, Hawaii and California. *J Stud Alcohol* **53**, 33–39.
21. Kim, S., McLeod, J.H. and Shantzis, C. (1992) Cultural competence for evaluators working with Asian-American communities: Some practical considerations, in *Cultural Competence for Evaluators: A Guide for Alcohol and Other Drug Abuse Prevention Practitioners Working with Ethnic/Racial Communities* (eds M.A Orlandi, R. Weston and L.G. Epstein), Rockville, MD: US Dept of Health and Human Services, Office forf Substance Abuse Prevention, pp. 203–260.
22. Furuto, S.M., Biswas, R., Chung, D.K., Murase, K. and Ross-Sheriff, F. (1992) *Social Work Practice with Asian Americans*, Sage: Thousand Oaks, CA.
23. Tanjasiri, S.P., Wallace, S.P. and Shibata, K. (1995) Picture imperfect: Hidden problems among Asian Pacific Islanders elderly. *The Gerontologist* **35**, 753–760.
24. Uehara, E.S., Takeuchi, D.T. and Smukler, M. (1994) Effects of combining disparate groups in the analysis of ethnic differences: Variations among Asian American

mental health consumers in level of functioning. *Am J Community Psychol.* **22**, 83–99.

25. Surgeon General. (1998) Tobacco use among US racial/ethnic minority groups: US Department of Health and Human Services. Center for Disease Control and Prevention.

26. Chi, I., Lubben, J.E. and Kitano, H.H.L. (1989) Differences in drinking behavior among three Asian-American groups. *J Stud Alcohol* **50**, 15–23.

27. Kitano, H.H.L. and Chi, I. (1988) Asian Americans and alcohol: The Chinese, Japanese, Koreans and Filipinos in Los Angeles, in *Alcohol Use Among US Ethnic Minorities* (eds D. Speigler. D. Tate, S. Aitken and C. Christian), National Institute on Alcohol and Alcohol Abuse: Rockville, MD.

28. Cassanelli, L.V.(1986) Qat: Changes in the production and consumption of a quasi-legal commodity in Northeast Africa, in *The Social Life of Things: Commodities in Cultural Perspective* (ed. A. Appadurai), Cambridge University Press: New York.

29. Hunt, G. and Barker, J.C. (1999) Drug treatment in contemporary anthropology and sociology. *Eur Addict Res.* **5**, 126–132.

30. Fabrega, H. and Manning, P.K. (1972) Disease, illness and deviant careers, in *Theoretical Perspectives on Deviance* (eds R.A. Scott and J.D. Douglas), Basic Books: New York.

31. Sinha, S.N. and Sengupta, S.K. (1989) Road traffic fatalities in Port Moresby: A ten year survey. *Accid Anal Prev.* **21**, 297–301.

32. Hunt, G. and Rosenbaum, M. (1998) 'Hustling' within the clinic: Consumer perspectives on methadone maintenance treatment, in *Heroin in the Age of Crack Cocaine* (eds J.A. Incicardi and L.D. Harrison), Sage: Thousand Oaks, CA.

33. Csordas, T.J. (ed.) (1994) *Embodiment and Experience: The Existential Ground of Culture and Self,* Cambridge University Press, New York.

34. Jenkins, J.H. (1996) Culture, emotion and psychiatric disorder, in *Medical Anthropology: Contemporary Theory and Method* (eds C.F. Sargent and T.M. Johnson), revised edition, Westport, CT: Praeger.

35. MacAndrew, C. and Edgerton, R. (1969) *Drunken Comportment: A Social Explanation,* Aldine: Chicago.

36. Beyene, Y. (1992) Medical disclosure and refugees: Telling bad news to Ethiopian patients. *West J Med.* **157**, 328–332.

37. Colsher, P.L., Wallace, R.B. and Pomrehn, P.R. and La Croix, A.Z. (1990) Demographic and health characteristics of elderly smokers: Results from established populations for epidemiologic studies of the elderly. *Am J Prev Med.* **6**, 61–70.

38. Barker, J.C. and Kramer, B.J. (1996) Alcohol consumption among older urban American Indians. *J Stud Alcohol* **57**, 119–124.

39. Blomqvist, J. (1996) Paths to recovery from substance misuse: Change of lifestyle and the role of treatment. *Subst Use Misuse* **31**, 1807–1852.

40. Klingemann, H. and Klingemann, H.-D. (1999) National treatment systems in global perspective. *Eur Addict Res.* **5**, 109–117.

41. MacGregor, S. (1999) Drug treatment systems and policy frameworks: A comparative social perspective. *Eur Addict Res.* **5**, 119–125.

42. Konuma, K., Shimizu, S. and Koyanagi, T. (1998) Social control and the model of legal drug treatment: A Japanese success story?, in *Drug Treatment Sustems in an International Perspective: Drugs, Demons and Delinquents* (eds H. Klingemann and G. Hunt), Sage: Thousand Oaks, CA.

43. Chin, S.-Y. (1992) This, that and the other – Managing illness in a first-generation Korean-American family. *West J Med.* **157**, 305–309.

44. Lara-Ponce, A. (1998) Who is to blame? The discovery of domestic drug problems and the quest for recognition of therapeutic communities in Peru, in *Drug*

Treatment Systems in an International Perspective: Drugs, Demons and Delinquents (eds H. Klingemann and G. Hunt), Sage: Thousand Oaks, CA.

45. Lewis, I.M. (1971) *Ecstatic Religion: An Anthropological Study of Spirit Possession and Shamanism*, Penguin: Harmondsworth.
46. Hellman, C. (1986) *Culture, Health and Illness*, Wright: Bristol.

Chapter eleven

Concluding comments: what I would tell my neighbor

NATURAL RECOVERY RESEARCH 'MATURING OUT'

This book and the literature it reviews show the broad range and impressive development of research into the self-change process over the past decade. In particular, general population studies have shown that self-change is a major pathway to recovery. This last chapter draws together the core findings and tailors them into a 'What I would tell my neighbor' format.

CREATING A SOCIETAL CLIMATE FRIENDLY TO INDIVIDUAL CHANGE: ADVICE FOR POLICY-MAKERS

Many individuals who have had problems with alcohol, drugs, tobacco, and gambling solve them without treatment. However, most people are not aware that such recovery occurs [1]. In this regard, efforts are needed to increase awareness among the general public that many people with addictive behavior can change on their own. Increased awareness may also make it easier for friends and relatives to encourage substance abusers to stop or reduce their use.

The frequent occurrence of self-change coupled with the general public's lack of awareness of such recovery suggests that disseminating knowledge about the prevalence of self-change would itself be a type of intervention. Individuals who have achieved such recovery could make public declarations in order to help others consider engaging in the self-change process. Some effort should also be made to inform substance abusers about the possibility that others can aid their recovery by being supportive. Self-help manuals should be widely available and should inform individuals with addictive behavior that they can recover without professional treatment [2].

Public health and education campaigns like those described in Chapter 9 can be an effective means of raising public awareness. An example is community interventions in which, rather than targeting individuals for change efforts, the targets are opinion leaders, medical practitioners, or public health officials.

191

Community-oriented interventions should be developed, including both information campaigns and the establishement of treatment-umbrella or resource-umbrella organizations that assist individuals to function and to address specific problems.

More specifically, natural contact points need to be identified for disseminating information on behavior change/health information and 'teachable moments' (e.g. medical-visit waiting time, pharmacists as credible reference sources). In addition, Internet health advice and expert systems should be made accessible to large segments of the population. Such policy interventions in turn are likely to trigger and facilitate change at the grass roots (e.g. Mothers against Drunk Driving; Moderation Management, a self-help group for problem drinkers who did not feel comfortable with traditional self-help groups such as Alcoholics Anonymous).

BARRIERS TO PUTTING POLICY ADVICE INTO PRACTICE

Attempts to implement advice for policy makers may evoke opposition. For example, those that might be opposed to such advice are pharmaceutical companies marketing smoking-cessation products, groups seeking more recognition and treatment for recently recognized addiction problems (e.g. gambling), advocates of traditional substance-abuse treatment. In the USA for example, opposition may come from an extremely activist drug czar, Congress, and Partnership for a Drug Free America, all of whom have defined as a national priority the elimination of drug use. Strategies will be needed to (a) overcome resistance, (b) build coalitions, and (c) support policies derived from self-change research.

SELF-CHANGE AND TREATMENT: STRIKING THE RIGHT BALANCE

The treatment industry will not necessarily oppose the idea of self-change, because prompting substance abusers to attempt self-change can also lead to involving them more in treatment. This would be consistent with current trends in the treatment system. Peele [3] has argued that we are in the midst of a tremendous 'treatment splurge'. When treatment of substance abuse expands, the natural direction for this expansion is to less severely dependent individuals, because such individuals are more amenable to change, more appealing to deal with, and better able to pay for treatment than those who are more severely dependent. Sobell and Sobell [4] have described intermediate forms of treatment such as 'Guided Self-Change' for this population. However, unless the treatment system in the US is radically remodeled (for example, it is almost completely abstinence-oriented), attracting less severely impaired users into treatment will continue to be a problem. In traditional programs such users are typically required to acknowledge they are substance abusers, and that they are addicted. Those who refuse to label themselves are accused of being in 'denial'.

When we consider research on gamblers who change on their own but do not see themselves as having had a problem (see Chapter 4, ref. 12), we may detect a paradoxical effect from so-called denial. That is, for a sizable proportion of natural recoveries, the process of change takes into account, and may even be based on, the refusal to label oneself as having a severe addiction.

It should be kept in mind when advocating self-change that people must not be discouraged from seeking treatment when they need it. Some substance abusers may not be able to recover without treatment and we do not want to reduce the likelihood that they will be able to receive treatment. In addition, learning about barriers to treatment and making specific types of treatment more accessible and acceptable for under-served populations (e.g. HIV + substance abuser; women) should not lead to an artificial expansion of the treatment industry. Any efforts to change beliefs about the extent of self-directed recovery versus professional treatment should be introduced prudently and monitored to be sure that the efforts are not discouraging people from entering treatment or self-help groups. Also, clinicians tend to see people struggling to change. But, when the frame of reference shifts to large groups of people, we see instead that people are all the time shifting back and forth across boundaries of 'problems' or 'addictions', seemingly effortlessly or without forethought. Of course, we realize much goes into these 'effortless changes', both at the individual and at the environmental/social level, which this book tries to make clear.

ADVICE FOR TREATMENT PROVIDERS

The evidence resulting from self-change research presented in this book endorses the concept of *stepped care* (see Chapter 6). It is based on a view of recovery that considers routes of change ranging from self-change to assisted self-change (e.g. bibliotherapy) to guided self-change (e.g. brief interventions, discussions with physicians) to more intensive outpatient and inpatient treatments.

For self-change or assisted self-change choice and diversity need to be provided, including harm reduction approaches. These efforts are likely to encounter resistance from those who hold traditional views, because outcomes in which addicts do not cease drug use will not be viewed as acceptable. Harm reduction programs (e.g. needle exchange or the substitution of oral opioids for injected drugs, server training for bar-keepers and drinking guidelines) are intended to minimize health problems, without necessarily resolving the addiction [5]. Nonetheless, harm reduction programs improve people's lives [6]. Harm reduction should be considered improvement, and such a transition may be a precursor over the long run to a more fully remitted state.

More important than increased levels of treatment is the shift in intervention modalities and structure suggested by natural-recovery data. Among the changes in treatment that follow from the recognition of the frequent occurrence of natural recoveries are the following:

- Language used by health care practitioners with their clients needs to change. Such terms as 'addict' and 'alcoholic' carry stigma. Not only is there no clinical advantage to labeling, but also it leads to reluctance to seek or enter treatment. Motivational interviewing teaches us how to approach clients to increase their readiness to change or to strengthen their commitment to change [7]. Along these same lines, interventions should be designed to have consumer appeal [2, 8].

- Interventions need to be flexible so that they can focus on improved functioning as well as on cessation of substance use.

- Gradual improvements in a person's addictive career, and particularly non-abstinence outcomes, should be important, acceptable, and documented aspects of treatment.

- Self-change outcomes and methods should be well publicized.

IMPROVING THE BASIS FOR EVIDENCE-BASED POLICIES: ADVICE FOR THE RESEARCH COMMUNITY

Methodological groundwork for research into the process of self-change needs to be improved in the following ways:

- Prospective studies are needed that help answer questions of causal relationships, and for a better integration of qualitative and quantitative approaches.

- Improvements in methodological design are needed, such as the use of control groups, validity tests using interviews with collaterals, and the development of standardized instruments to measure self-change over time [9].

- Studies of addictive-behavior change need to link verbal reports to observational data. We need to keep in mind that the illusion of control favors attributions to temporally contiguous 'causes' – so-called of 'telling more than we can know'.

- A comparison within the same research design of self-identified self-changers with those identified by 'objective' (survey past and present) assessments – since the former almost resemble treated changers, while the latter may be completely unaware of their change.

Future applied research needs to be focused on the following substantive topics:

- Comparative studies that include in a single research design various problem areas, particularly licit and illicit drugs as well as eating disorders, medication misuse, and addiction unrelated to substance use.

- Increased attention to the social contextual factors, 'social capital,' and social response to natural recovery that ultimately affect the chances of sustained self-change. With social empowerment, more people are likely to want or to be able to change. The research indicates that these are the primary environmental dimensions that permit change – personal opportunity, economic well-being, absence of stress, social support, and social values that encourage moderate behavior or abstinence in the area of concern.

- The investigation of change processes in different cultural contexts.

- A better understanding of drifting out of problems 'without any reason'.

- Research that combines cross-sectional research designs with in-depth qualitative methods has great potential for advancing knowledge about self-change.

- Studies on the process of change in addictive behavior among persons with different help-seeking experiences would be helpful because it may be possible to relate etiological processes to routes of change and care-seeking.

- Studies on the role of spiritual factors in natural recovery studies, such as 'legal highs' (e.g. sensation seeking, religious experiences).

- Natural experiments of social contextual capitalizing upon natural recovery events such as local disasters as well as legal changes such as modifications of gambling regulations and smoking restrictions in public places.

CONCLUSIONS

Scientists have to remove their research hats occasionally and take an active part in shaping policy on addictive behavior. Although changing public images of addiction can be an objective for scientists, they must be knowledgeable and skillful in their interactions with the media. Visible research networks can be used to bring science to the public. The examples of media campaigns based on empirical findings from the self-change literature indicate that science can influence policy. For example, social scientists working together with policy-makers within the framework of the Swiss National Alcohol Action Plan (which in turn was based on a WHO initiative) have successfully 'marketed' their ideas.

In addition, it is critical that scientists and health care providers learn to interact with, and learn from, each other [10]. Implementing brief interventions in practice and studying the solutions and coping strategies that successful self-changers use is essential. Meetings such as that held in September 2000 in Lausanne, Switzerland, at which the medical community met the scientific community on the topic of 'brief interventions', can serve as a vehicle for the dissemination of what is known in this area.

In terms of knowledge management, self-change research needs to be connected with treatment and political systems. So far, advice presented has been segmented for policy, treatment, and science. These areas need to be networked with action based on the concerns of multiple stakeholders. This book and the conference upon which it has been based represents (a) actualizing an interdisciplinary approach to understanding the self-change process, and (b) an early step towards facilitating communication among scientists, policy-makers, and health care practitioners from different schools of thought.

REFERENCES

1. Cunningham, J.A., Sobell, L.C. and Sobell, M.B. (1998) Awareness of self-change as a pathway to recovery for alcohol abusers: Results from five different groups. *Addict Behav.* 23(3), 399–404.
2. Peele, S., Brodsky, A. and Arnold, W.M. (1991) *The Truth About Addiction and Recovery: The Life Process Program for Outgrowing Destructive Habits*, Simon and Schuster: New York.
3. Peele, S. (1989) *Diseasing of America: Addiction Treatment Out of Control*, Lexington Books: Lexington, MA.
4. Sobell, M.B. and Sobell, L.C. (1993) *Problem Drinkers: Guided Self-Change Treatment*, Guilford Press: New York.
5. DesJarlais, D.C. (1995) Harm reduction: A framework for incorporating science into drug policy. *Am J Public Health* 85, 10–12.
6. Marlatt, G.A. (1998) *Harm Reduction: Pragmatic Strategies for Managing High-Risk Behaviors*, Guilford Press: New York.
7. Substance Abuse and Mental Health Administration. (1999) Enhancing motivation for change in substance abuse treatment (Treatment Improvement Protocol Series No. 35). U.S. Department of Health and Human Services: Rockville, MD.
8. Sobell, M.B. and Sobell, L.C. (1998) Guiding self-change, in *Treating Addictive Behaviors*, 2nd edn (eds W.R. Miller and N. Heather), Plenum: New York, pp. 189–202.
9. Sobell, L.C., Ellingstad, T.P. and Sobell, M.B. (2000) Natural recovery from alcohol and drug problems: Methodological review of the research with suggestions for future directions. *Addiction* 95, 749–769.
10. Sobell, L.C. (1996) Bridging the gap between scientists and practitioners: The challenge before us. *Behav Ther.* 27(3), 297–320.

Self-change toolbox: tools, tips, and other information and resources for assisting self-change

INTRODUCTION

This toolbox is intended to provide tools, tips and other information and resources to assist and promote the self-change process. Included in this toolbox is a listing of brief assessment instruments, an extensive listing of addictive behavior websites by different countries, as well as a selective listing of self-change books, videos, resources guides and articles, also by country.

It was not the intention of the authors to have an inclusive listing of self-change tools, tips and resources. Rather, the selection of items reflects the preferences and experiences of the authors as well as those of several other contributors, including the following: F. Beccaria (Italy), E. Dallolio (Great Britain), N. Heather (Great Britain), A. Koski-Jännes (Finland), H. Kuefner (Germany), and H.-J. Rumpf (Germany).

ASSESSMENT INSTRUMENTS TO FACILITATE SELF-CHANGE

There is no shortage of instruments for assessing addictive behavior [1–8]. This toolbox lists and describes, in most cases brief instruments that can be used to facilitate and evaluate the self-change process. The criteria for choosing the instruments were that they were brief, required minimal time and resources, and were readily accessible and free. When choosing an instrument for use in facilitating self-change, it should, whenever possible, provide meaningful advice/feedback that can enhance or strengthen motivation for change [8].

The use of brief measures [9–15] has increased dramatically over the past decade, spurred on by self-change andbrief interventions [16–20]. Thus, while the Addiction Severity Index (ASI), for example, has excellent psychometric characteristics [21] and has been used in many drug programs [21], it is a structured interview with 147 questions (assesses problems in seven different areas) that must be administered by a trained interviewer and it takes about 30 to 45 minutes. Consequently, such instruments are too labor-intensive and demand too many resources for use in a brief self-change intervention that can be as little as one session.

ASSESSING PROBLEM SEVERITY OR ADVERSE CONSEQUENCES

Alcohol use disorders identification test (AUDIT)

A 10-item self-administered questionnaire. Addresses past and recent alcohol consumption and alcohol-related problems; it takes 3–5 minutes to complete and it identifies individuals drinking at high risk levels as well as those already experiencing consequences [1, 22, 23]. Available in English, French, Spanish, Portuguese and German.

Drug abuse screening test (DAST)

A 10-item self-administered questionnaire measuring drug consequences that occurred in the last year; it takes 3–5 minutes to complete [2, 5, 24]. Available in English, Spanish and Portuguese.

Lübeck alcohol dependence and abuse screening test (LAST)

A 7-item short questionnaire which screens for alcohol dependence and abuse. It takes about 1–2 minutes to complete. The questionnaire is especially suited for use in health care settings [25].

South Oaks gambling screen (SOGS)

A 20-item self-administered questionnaire. Assesses gambling-related consequences that have occurred over the person's lifetime; it takes 3–5 minutes to complete [26].

Time to the first cigarette

While a nicotine-dependence score is useful for research purposes, clinically one question is useful – 'How many minutes upon waking until the first cigarette is smoked?' The latency interval to smoking the first cigarette after waking is strongly predictive of nicotine dependence [27]. This question is part of the Fagerström scale for assessing nicotine dependence [28].

ASSESSING ALCOHOL, DRUGS, SMOKING OR GAMBLING

Drug use history questionnaire (DUHQ)

The DUHQ captures lifetime and recent information (e.g. years used, route of administration, year last used, frequency of use) about the use of different drugs. It uses a card-sort technique and takes 5–10 minutes to complete [15, 29].

One alcohol question

Three studies have found that a single question such as 'Have you ever had a drinking problem' results in the identification of more individuals as having an alcohol problem than more complex screening tests, such as the Michigan Alcohol Screening Test [29–32].

Self-monitoring

Self-monitoring requires clients to record aspects (e.g. amount, frequency, mood, urges) of their addictive behavior (e.g. alcohol, drug, smoking, gambling) throughout treatment. Self-monitoring has several clinical uses: (a) it helps clients to be continually aware of their substance use or other addictive behavior, and safeguards against distorted perceptions of use; (b) it provides a picture of the client's addictive behavior during treatment; (c) it identifies situations that pose a high risk of use and relapse; (d) it provides a basis for evaluating whether a change in the target behavior is occurring; and (e) it gives clients an opportunity to talk without awkwardness about their addictive behavior with their therapist during treatment [14, 15, 30].

ASSESSING HIGH RISK TRIGGERS TO ADDICTIVE BEHAVIOR

Brief SCQ-8 (BSCQ)

Because addictive behavior has a high rate of relapse it is essential to evaluate high-risk triggers to use during an intervention [35]. The BSCQ, a variant of the Situational Confidence Questionnaire [1, 34], asks about eight major categories of situations related to alcohol or drug use [9]. Unlike the SCQ, the BSCQ is easy to score, can be used to provide immediate feedback to clients about high-risk triggers to their alcohol or drug use, and is free [8, 9]. A similar brief instrument has recently been developed for gamblers [36].

ASSESSING MOTIVATION/READINESS TO CHANGE

There has been an increasing recognition of the importance of assessing the extent to which individuals with addictive behavior believe change is necessary [8]. Motivation can be conceptualized as a state of readiness to change that may fluctuate over time and can be influenced by several things, including the health care practitioner [8]. The important issue for health care practitioners is that interventions for individuals who are not strongly committed to changing their addictive behavior should initially focus on increasing their motivation, rather than on methods of changing.

Decisional balancing exercise

This exercise asks clients to evaluate their perceptions of the costs and benefits of continuing to engage in addictive behavior versus changing; it is intended to make more salient the costs and benefits of changing and to identify obstacles to change [37–39]. Copies of a Decisional Balance Exercise can be found in a recent publication on motivational interviewing [8].

Interviewing style

Interviewing style is very important for obtaining accurate information about a person's substance use. The way questions are asked can affect a person's answers. An important part of motivational interviewing is to avoid labeling. Individuals with substance-use problems are generally reluctant to be labeled as an 'alcoholic' or a 'drug addict', and this particularly applies to individuals whose problems are not severe. Labeling should be avoided because it has no advantages, and because it has been associated with substance abusers delaying or avoiding entry to treatment [40–42]. Asking people with an alcohol or drug problem to 'tell me about your use in the past year and any concerns you may have' is more likely to get them to engage in an open dialogue about their use than asking them 'How long have you been an alcoholic (or drug addict)'? The following two references provide examples of how to ask the right questions [8, 43].

Motivational strategies and procedures to increase motivation

(a) help individuals identify discrepancies between their goals and their current behavior;
(b) help individuals identify reasons for changing;
(c) enhance individuals' reasons for change by providing feedback on the risks and consequences of their behavior; and
(d) help individuals develop and evaluate plans for changing.

Socrates

The Stage Of Change Readiness and Treatment Easiness Scale (SOCRATES) is a 19-item scale to assess motivation for change with alcohol abusers [44].

ADDICTION SELF-CHANGE WEBSITES BY COUNTRY

North America

Alcoholics Anonymous: < http://www.alcoholics-anonymous.org >
Canadian Centre on Substance Abuse: < www.ccsa.ca >
Canadian Foundation on Compulsive Gambling: < www.responsiblegambling. org >
Free self-help material and free self-monitoring software:
< www.behaviortherapy,com >
Habit Smart: < www.cts.com/crash/habtsmrt > provides a broad range of self-help information.
Moderation Management: < http://www.moderation.org >
Rational Recovery: < http://www.rational.org/recovery >
Smart Recovery: < http://www.smartrecovery.org >
Stanton Peele Addiction Web-Site: < http://www.peele.net > offers non-traditional and natural remission perspective on variety of addictions.
Web of Addictions: (link page) < http://www.well.com/user/woa >
Addiction Severity Index: Manual and tape. Order No. AVA Delta Metrics TRJ 19615VNB2, National Technical Information Services. Tel: 703-487-4650 or 800-238-2433.
Brown University Center for Alcohol and Addiction Studies: Curriculum and training materials for health care professionals. Brown University, Box G-BH, Providence, RI 02912. Tel: 401-863-1000.
Cancer Prevention Research Center at the University of Rhode Island: < www.uri.edu/research/cprc > instruments to assess stages and processes of change (alcohol and smoking) as well as related constructs (decisional balance, self-efficacy). Information on the Transtheoretical Model of Change.
Center on Alcoholism, Substance Abuse and Addictions:
< wrmiller@unm-edu > motivational interviewing articles and tapes; W.R. Miller. Department of Psychology, University of New Mexico, Albuquerque, NM, 87131-1161.
Centre for Addiction and Mental Health: (formerly the Addiction Research Foundation). < www.camh.net >. Assessment and treatment planning tools. 33 Russell St., Toronto, Ontario, M5S 2S1, Canada. Tel: 800-661-1111.

Center for Online-Addiction: <www.netaddiction.com/> information about Internet addiction, addiction tests, online counselling, book presentations and press reviews in English.

Guided Self-Change Clinic: <www.nova.edu/~gsu> <sobell@nova.edu> Timeline Followback materials and other Guided Self-Change materials and forms; L. C. Sobell. Center for Psychological Studies, Nova Southeastern University, 3301 College Ave., Ft. Lauderdale, FL 33314.

Higher Education Center for Alcohol and Other Drug Prevention: <http://www.edc.org/hec> provides access to databases as well as other information about effective substance abuse prevention programs; public policy options; substance abuse educational opportunities for parents, students and community leaders; and publications.

Motivational Interviewing: <www.motivationalinterview.org> this site serves as a resource for organizations who seek training in motivational interviewing. (The site also contains links to other useful websites).

National Clearinghouse Alcohol and Drug Information:
<http://www.health.org> <telnet:ncadi.health.org> <ftp.health.org> <info@prevline.health.org> PO Box 2345. Rockville, MD 20852, USA. Tel: 301-468-2600, 1-800-729-6686. The information service of the Center for Substance Abuse Prevention of the USDHHS. It serves as the central point in the Federal Government for information about alcohol and other drug problems. Many of its publications can be obtained free of charge by calling the toll free number and providing one's name and address. Items are also available on line for downloading.

National Institute on Alcohol Abuse and Alcoholism: <www.niaaa.nih.gov> <http://etoh.niaaa.nih.gov> (literature search program); 6000 Executive Blvd, Rockville, Maryland 20892-7003.

National Institute on Drug Abuse: <www.nida.nih.gov> NIDA infofax: Science based facts on drug abuse and addiction. Tel: 1-888-644-6432 (free fact sheets).

NIDA-supported Monitoring the Future Study: <http://www.isr.umich.edu/src/mtf> provides data on the prevalence and trends in drug use among American high school students and young adults.

Rutgers University Center of Alcohol Studies: Large collection of alcohol information. Smithers Hall, Busch Campus, Piscataway, NH, 08855-0969. Tel: 908-445-2190.

Smoking Websites:
<www.tobacco.org>
<www.tobacco.org/History/Tobacco_History.html>
<www.kickbutt.org> (Smoking Cessation Facts)
<www.lungusa.org> (American Lung Association);
<wwwonder.cdc.gov> (CDC Prevention Guidelines;
<www.clc.upmc.edu/CLC_HTML/smoking.htm> (Smoking Cessation Behavior Modification);

<www.welltech.com/netconnect/smoke.html> (Smoking Cessation Resources);

<www.ahcpr.gov> (Smoking Cessation Clinical Practice Guideline; free, published by Agency for Health Care Policy and Research. Tel: 800-358-9295).

Great Britain

The Advisory Council on Alcohol and Drug Education (TACADE): <www.tacade.com> aims to provide support for professional groups working with young people. Provides a range of publications and training products. 1 Hulme Place, Salford, Manchester, M5 4QA. Tel: 0161-745-8925.

Alcohol Concern: <www.alcoholconcern.org.uk> a national agency on alcohol use. Its website contains a vast amount of information about the effects of drinking. The site includes a page of local contact points and links to other alcohol-related sites. 32–36 Loman Street, London SE1 0EE. Tel: 020-7928-7377.

Alcohol Problem Advisory Service: <www.apas.org.uk> offers information, training and advice on alcohol misuse. 36 Park Row, Nottingham NG1 6GR. Tel: 0115-948-5570.

Centre for Health Economics: <www.york.ac.uk/inst/che> A central point for alcohol information and trends. University of York, Heslington, York YO1 5DD. Tel: 01904-433-646.

Department of Health: <www.doh.gov.uk> provides statistics and information on alcohol use and misuse. Government reports and official documents can be obtained via the website. Richmond House, 79 Whitehall, London, SW1A 2NL. Tel: 020-7210-4850.

Institute of Alcohol Studies: <www.ias.org.uk> aims at increasing knowledge of alcohol misuse. Its website has a range of factsheets and publications related to alcohol issues. In addition, in the Medical Education section, it contains information on the knowledge and skills doctors need in order to identify and treat alcohol problems. Alliance House, 12 Caxton Street, London, SW1H 0QS. Tel: 020-7222-4001.

Jeff Allison: <www.jeffallison.co.uk> experienced trainer in motivational interviewing techniques, training courses available.

Medical Council on Alcoholism (MCA): <www.mca.medicouncilalcol.demon.co.uk> has an education and advisory role within the medical profession. Produces handbooks and newsletters and its website contains links to further resources. 3 St Andrew's Place, London, NW1 4LB. Tel: 020-7487-4445.

Motivational interviewing and smoking: <www.wcsquare.demon.co.uk/training/motiv/htm>

National Institute for Clinical Excellence: <www.nice.org.uk> contains information on behavioral changes and the benefits of motivational interviewing. Support for doctors, nurses and other health professionals. 90 Long Acre, Covent Garden, London, WC2E 9RZ. Tel: 020-7849-3444.

NHS Direct: <www.nhsdirect.nhs.uk> information, advice and details on support groups for health issues such as alcohol and smoking. Tel: 0845-4647.

Training by Distance Learning: <training@lau.org.uk> the course offers extensive teaching materials, weekly telephone tutorials with an experienced practitioner and also video-linked supervised practice. Leeds Addiction Unit, 19 Springfield Mount, Leeds, LS2, 9NG. Tel: 0113-295-1330.

Wrecked: think about drink: <www.wrecked.co.uk>

Smoking Websites:
<www.ash.org.uk>
<www.cancernet.co.uk/smoking.htm>
<http://healthnet.org.uk/quit/guide.htm>
<http://givingupsmoking.co.uk> – also offers free publication material
<www.nicotine-anonymous.org>
<www.recovery.org.uk>

Germany

AA Anonyme Alkoholiker Deutschland: <www.anonyme-alkoholiker.de> offizielle Homepage der AA in Deutschland. Viele Seiten sind noch im Aufbau; daher gibt es noch kaum Informationen, die nicht auch auf andern Seiten erhältlich sind.

AA Intergroup: <http://aa-intregroup.org> Diskussionsgruppen online: Mailinglisten und Chatgroups. Es gibt Gruppen in zahlreichen Sprachen – Mailinglisten (aber keine Chats) auch in Deutsch.

AA Online: <www.aa-online.de> zahlreiche weitere Internet – Diskussionsgruppen und zwar alle in deutscher Sprache.

Bücherliste Thema Essstörungen: <http://team.solution.de/gsf/selbsthilfe/cinderella/buecher.html>

Bulimie-Online: <www.bulimie-online.de>

Bundesministerium für Gesundheit: <www.bmgesundheit.de> (German Health Ministry) sehr ansprechend gestaltete Homepage des Ministeriums, welche auch für die deutsche Suchtmittelpolitik verantwortlich zeichnet. Neben zahlreichen aktuellen Texten findet man eine effektive Suchmaschine, einen attraktiv gestalteten Rundgang durch das Ministerium und interaktive Angebote.

Cinderella: <http://team.solution.de/gsf/selbshilfe/cinderella> Selbsthilfe-Dislussionsforum in Echtzeit (Chat) und zeitverschoben. Zusätzlich werden Leidens- und Lebensgeschichten und zahlreiche weitere interessante Informationen geboten.

Deutsche Gesellschaft für Suchtforschung und Suchttherapie e.V.: < www.psy. uni-muenster.de/institut1/dgs/dg-sucht > < dg-sucht@t-online.de > (German Society for addiction research and therapy). Interdiziplinäre Gesellschaft für Experten im Suchtbereich. U.a. Entwicklung von Dokumentationsstandards für die Durchfphrung von Evaluationsstudien im Suchtbereich. Alle 2 Jahre Veranstaltung einer zentralen wissenschaftlichen Veranstaltung über Sucht in Deutschland. Tel: 02381-417998.

Deutsche Hauptstelle gegen die Suchtgefahren: < www.dhs.de > (German organization against addiction dangers). Dachorganisation aller nicht privaten Verbände, die im Suchtbereich tätig sind. Informationen über Behandlungsplätze, Mitgliedsverbände und zahlreiche Links zu den wichtigsten anderen Organisationen im Suchtbereich. Organisation von Tagungen im Suchtbereich. Herausgeber der jährlich publizierten Reihe: DHS (Hrsg.): Jahrbuch Sucht Geesthacht: 2000 mit allen witchtigen Adressen von Organisationen sowie Berichten über neueste epidemiologische Zahlen und Entwicklungen im Suchtbereich. Tel: 02381-90150.

Deutsche Referenzstelle für die Europäische Beobachtungsstelle für Drogen und Drogensucht: < www.DBDD.de > (German reference for the European drugs and drug addiction observation group) Ansprechpartner für Fragen aus dem Bereich Epidemiologie der Sucht und Nachfragereduzierung.

Fachverband Glücksspielsucht e.V.: < www.gluecksspielsucht.de > Tel: 05221-599850. Für Informationen speziell über pathologisches Spielen.

Fachverband Sucht e.V.: < www.sucht.de > Tel: 0228-261555. Verband privater Einrichtungen zur Suchttherapie. Herausgeber einer eigenen Zeitschrift Sucht aktuell. Veranstalter eines järlicher Fachkongresses.

Fachverbank Drogen und Rauschmittel. e.V.: < www.neuland.com/fdr > Verband von therapeutischen Einrichtungen, die hauptsächlich im Bereich illegaler Drogen tätig sind. Tel: 0511-18333.

Hilfe zur Selbsthilfe für Online-Süchtige: < www.onlinesucht.de > Beratung, Selbsthilfegruppen, Mailinglisten, Interviews zum Thema, Online-Umfrage, Pressemitteilungen und wissenschaftliche Erkenntnisse.

Hungrig-Online: < www.hungrig-online.de > Foren, Mailingliste und Chat zum Thema. Die Seite ist die Diskussionsplattform der Informationsseiten Magersucht-online und Bulimie-Online.

Magersucht-Online: < www.magersucht-online.de >

Streichholz: < www.streichholz.ev.de > Verein der Eltern und Angehörigen von Anorexie und Bulimie Erkrankten. Seite mit sehr knappen, leicht vertändlichen Informationen rund ums Thema. Ohne interaktives Forum.

Verhaltenstherapeutische Ausbildung im Bereich Sucht:
< www.vtausbildung.de > die verhaltenstherapeutisch orientierten Trainings werden vom Institut für Therapieforschung (IFT), München, durchgeführt.

Austria

AA Anonyme Alkoholiker Oesterreich: < www.anonyme-alkoholiker.at >
professionell gestaltete Seite, welche neben den üblichen Informationen
(siehe Schweiz) eine ausführliche Darstellung der Geschichte zur Entwicklung der AA in den USA und in Europa bietet.
Anorexia Nervosa (Oesterreich): < www.angkfunigraz.ac.at/ ~ trojovsk/doc/
anorexia.html >

Finland

Alcohol or other substance problem: < http://www.paihdelinkki.fi >
< www.elamantapaliitto.fi > Web page of a Lifestyle Association, which
organizes short term (4 sessions) groups for people who want to cut down
their drinking and self-help groups for people who misuse sleeping pills and
tranquilizers. This association also provides related information and
organizes various joint activities for people who want to improve their
lifestyle.
< www.health.fi > Web page on health-related services in Finland. Includes
also links to various sources of information on alcohol, legal and illegal
drugs, smoking, etc.

France

Everything you have always wanted to know about alcohol and alcoholism:
< www.alcoweb.com >

Italy

Alcolisti Anonimi in Italia: < http://www.alcolisti-anonimi.it >
Associazione Italiana Club degli Alcolisti in Trattamento: < http://www.ai-
cat.net >
Aliseo (association against alcoholism):
< http://www.gruppoabele.it/attivita/accoglienza/aliseo.html >
Gruppo Abele: < http://www.gruppoabele.it > central point for information
on drugs and alcohol and other social problems, also offers different kinds
of recovery.
DrogaNet: < http://www.droga.net > news, links, discussion on drugs.
Osservatorio sul tabacco – Istituto Italiano Tumori:
< http://www.istitutotumori.mi.it./osservatorio/tabacco4.htm > offers dif-
ferent solutions to stop smoking)
Why and how to give up smoking Lega Italiana per la lotta contro i tumori:
... to stop smoking, and other methods

Sweden

Centre for Evaluation of Social Work: <http://www.sos.se/sos/publ/skrift/ cusrapp.htm> Swedish version of the Addiction Severity Index.

National Institute of Public Health: <http://www.fhi.se/lankar> provides links to websites with facts and/or advice about drinking, smoking and gambling.

National Council for Information on Alcohol and Drugs (CAN): <http:// www.can.se> Facts and figures about alcohol and drugs, library services etc.

Swedish Council for Information on Alcohol and Other Drugs: <http:// www.can.se> provides links to a number of relevant organisations and authorities, publishes topical facts and has a rather extensive addiction library.

Psyk@socialt Forum: <http://www.sposit.se> Catalogue of links, covering the whole psychosocial sector, including alcohol and drug information.

Switzerland

Institut Suisse de Prévention de l'Alcoolisme et autres toxicomanies:
Schweizerische Fachstelle für Alkohol- und andere Drogenprobleme:
<www.sfa-ispa.ch> <info@sfa-ispa.ch> Av. Ruchonnet 14, 1001 Lausanne. Tel: 021-32129-11, Fax: 021-32129-40, (Organisation non-gouvernementale spécialisée dans les domaines de l'alcool, du tabac et des drogues illégales, avec départements de recherche et de prévention. Bibliothèque, informations et statistiques, service question-réponse, connections avec d'autres sources d'aide en Europe, développement d'actions de prévention, recherche psycho-sociale, travail de lobbying politique ainsi qu'avec les médias).

Infoset Direct: <www.infoset.ch> Kommunikations- und Informationsinstrument im Suchtbereich. Das Ziel von infoset direct ist, Fachleuten und Nicht-Fachleuten einen Ueberblick über die Suchtarbeit in der Schweiz zu vermitteln und die Vernetzung zu fördern.

Talk about – ein Präventionsprojekt zur Verringerung des Alkoholkonsums bei Jugendlichen: <www.talkabout.org> dieses Projekt der Suchtpräventionsstelle des Blauen Kreuzes Bern hat folgende Ziele: Verzögerung des Einstiegs in den Alkoholkonsum, Bestärkung von Nichtkonsumierenden, Sensibilisierung für einen bewussten Umgang mit der Droge Alkohol.

AA Anonyme Alkoholiker deutschsprachige Schweiz:
<www.anonyme-alkooholiker.ch> zahlreiche Kontaktadressen, ein Test zur Selbsteinschätzung des Alkoholkonsums, Literaturvorschläge, Geschichtliches, 12 Schritte der AA.

Allen Carr's Easyway Nichtraucher-Page: <www.allen-carr.ch> schweizer Version eines Blitzprogrammes zur Rauchentwöhnung: 'In 6 Stunden zum Nichtraucher!'. Daneben gibt es Berichte von Entwöhnten aund aktuelle Medienmitteilungen im Bereich Tabakmissbrauch.

Fachstelle für Schadenminderung im Drogenbereich: <www.infoset.ch/inst/oseo>

Internet Campaign on Smoking Cessation: <www.yourmilestone.ch> uses significant life events as personal turning points, was launched by the Swiss Cancer League, (available in French, German and Italian). For more information contact : MILESTONE, c/o cR Kommunikation AG, Mr. Stefan Batzli, Seefeldstr. 92, CH-8034 Zurich. Tel: 001-387-4082.

ADDICTION SELF-CHANGE BOOKS, VIDEOS, RESOURCE GUIDES AND ARTICLES: BY COUNTRY

North America

Ayala, H.E., Lopez, G.C., Echeverria, L. and Lara, M. (1998) *Manual de Autoayuda para Personas con Problemas en Su Forma de Beber*, National University of Mexico: Mexico City, Mexico.

Ayala, H.E., Echeverria, L., Sobell, L.C. (1998) Una alternativa de intervencin breve y temprana parabebedores problema en México (An early and brief intervention for problem drinkers in Mexico). *Acta Comportamentalia* **6**, 71–93.

Bell, A. and Rollnick, S. (1996) Motivational interviewing in practice: A structured approach, in *Treating Substance Abuse: Theory and Technique* (eds F. Rotgers, D.S. Keller and J. Morgenstern), Guilford: New York, pp. 266–285.

D'Onofrio, G., Bernstein, E. and Bernstein, J. (1997) The Emergency Physician and the Problem Drinker: Motivating Patients for Change (videotape). Massachusetts: Boston and Yale University. Marino & Company Production. Tel: 800-548-9491. (29 minute training video)

D'Onofrio, G., Bernstein, E. and Rollnick, S. (1996) Motivating patients for change: A brief strategy for negotiation, in *Case Studies in Emergency Room Medicine and the Health of the Public* (eds E. Bernstein and J. Bernstein), Jones and Bartlett: Boston, pp. 295–303.

Hester, R., Handmaker, N. and Daitz, B. (1997) Motivating Pregnant Women to Stop Drinking (videotape). Southwest Production: Albuquerque, NM. Tel: 505-342-2472. (17 minute training video).

Miller, W.R. and Rollnick, S. (1991) *Motivational Interviewing: Preparing People to Change Addictive Behavior*, Guilford: New York.

Miller, W.R. (1998) Enhancing motivation for change, in *Treating Addictive Behaviors* 2nd edn (eds W.R. Miller and N. Heather), Plenum: New York, pp. 121–132.

Peele, S., Brodsky, A. and Arnold, M. (1991) *The Truth About Addiction and Recovery: The Life Process Program for Outgrowing Destructive Habits*, Simon and Schuster: New York.

Rollnick, S. (1998) Readiness, importance, and confidence, in *Treating Addictive Behaviors* 2nd edn (eds W.R. Miller and N. Heather), Plenum: New York, pp. 49–60.

Sanchez-Craig, M. (1993) *DrinkWise. How to Quit Drinking or Cut Down.* Addiction Research Foundation: Toronto, Ontario, 2nd revised edn 1995.
Sobell, L.C. and Sobell, M.B. (1995) *Motivational Strategies for Promoting Self-Change: Dealing with Alcohol and Drug Problems. Instructional Training Video.* Centre for Addiction and Mental Health Services, Toronto, Canada, <www.camh.net>. Tel: 800-661-1111. (38 minute training video).
Sobell, M.B. and Sobell, L.C. (1993) *Problem Drinkers: Guided Self-Change Treatment,* Guilford: New York.
Sobell, M.B. and Sobell, L.C. (1998) Guiding self-change, in *Treating Addictive Behaviors* 2nd edn (eds W.R. Miller and N. Heather), Plenum: New York, pp. 189–202.
Substance Abuse and Mental Health Administration. (1999) *Enhancing motivation for change in substance abuse treatment (Treatment Improvement Protocol Series No. 35),* Department of Health and Human Services: Rockville, MD: U.S. (Excellent comprehensive guidebook on how to do motivational interviewing. Can be obtained free of charge from the National Clearinghouse for Alcohol and Drug Dependence by calling 1-800-729-6686 or 301-468-2600and asking for DHHS Publication No. SMA 99-3354).
Can also be viewed on-line: <http://text.nlm.nih.gov>

Great Britain

British Medical Association (1985) *Alcohol: Guidelines on Sensible Drinking.* BMJ Publishing Group: London, UK.
Cantopher, T. (1996) *Dying for a Drink,* The Book Guild. London. 130 pp. (Practical guide for heavy drinkers and involved professionals).
Colclough, B. (1994) *The Effective Way to Stop Drinking,* Penguin Books Ltd.
Fanning, P. *et al.* (1996) *The Addiction Workbook (A Step-by-Step Guide to Quitting Alcohol and Drugs),* New Harbinger Publications: Oakland.
Robertson, I. and Heather, N. (1986) *Let's Drink to Your Health! A Self-Help Guide to Sensible Drinking,* 2nd edition, British Psychological Society: Leicester, UK.
Carr, A. (1995) *The Only Way to Stop Smoking Permanently,* Penguin Books Ltd: London, UK.
Howell, K. (1996) *Stop Smoking,* Brain Sync: Great Britain (Cassette).
Raw, M. (2000) *Kick the Habit,* BBC Consumer Publishing (Books): London, UK.
Bien, T.H., Miller, W.R. and Tonigan, J.S.(1993) Motivational interviewing with alcohol outpatients, *Behav Cognitive Psychother.* 21, 347–356.
Butler, C., Rollnick, S., Cohen, D., Russel, I., Bachmann, M. and Stott, N. (1999) Motivational consulting versus brief advice for smokers in general practices: A randomized trail, *Br J Gen Pract.* 49, 165–171.
Gleeson, C., Memom, I., Milner, M. and Barnes, S. (1997) Smoking cessation in pregnancy: A multiple contact approach, *Br J Midwifery* 5, 551–554.
Handmaker, N. *et al.* (1999) Findings of a pilot study of motivational interviewing with pregnant drinkers, *J Stud Alcohol* 60, 285–287.
Kushner, P.R., Levison, W. and Miller, W.R. (1998) Motivational interviewing: When, when and why. *Patient Care* 32(14), 55–72.
Noonan, W.C. and Moyers, T.B. (1997) Motivational interviewing: A review, *J Subst Misuse* 2, 8–16.
Rollnick, S. *et al.* (1993). Methods for helping patients with behaviour change. *Br Med J.* 307, 188–190.
Samet, J.H., Rollnick, S. and Barnes, H. (1996) Beyond CAGE: A clinical approach after detection of substance abuse. *Arch Internal Med.* 156, 2287–2293.

Finland

Borg, S. and Johansson, K. (1990) Irti unilääkkeistä ja rauhoittavista aineista. Porvoo: WSOY.

Kauppi, T. (1993) *Jos ottaminen ottaa päähän.* Otava: Helsinki.

Koski-Jännes, A. (1986) *Kuinka paljon on lian paljon? Opas juomisen vähentäjile ja lopettajile.* Otava: Helsinki (How much is too much? A guide for those who want to cut down or stop drinking).

Koski-Jännes, A., Jussila, A. and Hänninen, V. (1998) *Miten riippuvuus voitetaan.* Otava: Helsinki (This book covers the results from the study on people who had overcome different addictions).

Koski-Jännes, A. (1998) Turning points in addiction careers: five case studies, *Journal of Substance Misuse* 3, 226–233.

Koski-Jännes, A. and Turner N. (1999) Factors influencing recovery from different addictions, *Addiction Research* 7(6), 469–492.

Hänninen, V. and Koski-Jännes, A. (1999) Narratives of recovery from addictive behaviours, *Addiction* 94(12), 1837–1848.

Selvis (1999). *Ehkäisevän päihdetyön ja päihdehuollon yhteystiedot.* Terveyden edistämisen keskus, TEK: in julkaisujal.

Puska, P., Urjanheimo, E.-L. and Ikävalko, R. (1995) Irti Tupakasta. Lopettajan opas. Helsinki: Otava.

Germany

Carr, A. (1999) *Carr's Erfolgsmethode – Endlich Nichtraucher!* Mosaik Verlag: München.

Sweden

Andersson, B. and Hilte, M. (1993) *Förändringens väg: självförståelse och strategier i frigörelsen från drogmissbruk.* Lund: Network for research in criminology and deviant behaviour at Lund University. (About change strategies in overcoming drug problems).

Blomqvist, J. (1996) Paths to recovery from substance misuse: Change of lifestyle and the role of treatment. *Subst Use Misuse* 31, 1807–1852.

Blomqvist, J. (1999) Treated and untreated recovery from alcohol misuse. Environmental influences and perceived reasons for change. *Subst Use Misuse* 34, 1371–1406.

Blomqvist, J. (in press) Recovery with and without treatment. A comparison of resolutions of alcohol and drug problems. *Addict Res.*

Blomqvist, J. (in press) *Att sluta med narkotika – med och utan behandling.* FoU-rapport. Socialtjänsten i Stockholm: Fou-enheten (On treated and untreated recoveries from drug problems).

Blomqvist, J. (1999) *Inte bara behandling – vägar ut ur alkoholmissbruket.* Bokförlaget Bjurner and Bruno: Vaxholm, (Compares, describes and discusses treated and untreated recoveries from alcohol problems, general features in the path to recovery, implications for health professionals)

Berglund, M., Andréasson, S., Bergmark, A., Oscarsson, L., Tengvald, K. and Öjehagen, A., 1996. *Dokumentation inom missbrukarvården.* Eskilstuna: CUS and Liber Förlag. (Presents and discusses tools for assessment of alcohol and drug problems).

Berglund, M. *et al.* (2000) *Behandling av alkoholproblem – en kunskapsöversikt.* Stockholm: CUS och Liber förlag. (Anthology on alcohol problems and treatment, initiated by the Centre for Evaluation of Social Work (CUS) at the National Board of Health and Welfare and including discussion of self-change.

Kristiansen, A. (2000) *Fri från narkotika*. Bokförlaget Bjurner och Bruno, Vaxholm. (Based on interviews with men and women who broke free from drug misuse).

Switzerland

Rihs, M. and Lotti, H. (1993) *Frei vom Rauchen – Gezielt aufhören und das Leben neu geniessen*, Hans Huber Verlag: Bern-Göttingen-Toronto-Seattle (order through Hans Huber Verlag, Länggassstr. 76, CH- Bern 9)

Allemann, P.I. (1997) *Strukturierte Kurzintervention bei Alkoholpatienten - ein Handbuch mit praktischen Uebungen*. Lausanne: Schweizerische Fachstelle für Alkohol und andere Drogenprobleme. (ISBN 2-88183-064-1, order through <Info@sfa-ispa. ch> Tel: 41-21-321-2935). (German adaptation of 'Guided Self-Change', L. and M. Sobell, Toronto: ARF)

REFERENCES

1. Allen, J.P. and Columbus, M. (1995) *Assessing Alcohol Problems: A Guide for Clinicians and Researchers*, Rockville, MD: National Institute on Alcohol Abuse and Alcoholism.
2. American Psychiatric Association (2000) *Handbook of Psychiatric Measures*, American Psychiatric Association: Washington, DC.
3. López Viets, V.C.L. and Miller, W.R. (1997) Treatment approaches for pathological gamblers. *Clin Psychol Rev.* **17** 689–702.
4. Rounsaville, B.J. *et al.* (1993) *Diagnostic Source Book of Drug Abuse Research and Treatment*, National Institute on Drug Abuse: Rockville, MD.
5. Sobell, L.C. *et al.* (1994) Behavioral assessment and treatment planning for alcohol, tobacco, and other drug problems: Current status with an emphasis on clinical application. *Behav Ther.* **25**, 533–580.
6. Substance Abuse and Mental Health Administration. (1993) *Screening and Assessment of Alcohol and Other Drug-Abusing Adolescents (Treatment Improvement Protocol Series 3)*. Department of Health and Human Services: Rockville, MD, U.S.
7. Substance Abuse and Mental Health Administration. (1995) *Assessment and Treatment of Patients with Coexisting Mental Illness and Alcohol and Other Drug Abuse (Treatment Improvement Protocol Series 9)*. Department of Health and Human Services: Rockville, MD, U.S.
8. Substance Abuse and Mental Health Administration. (1999) *Enhancing Motivation for Change in Substance Abuse Treatment (Treatment Improvement Protocol Series No. 35)*. Department of Health and Human Services: Rockville, MD, U.S.
9. Breslin, F.C. *et al.* (2000) A comparison of a brief and long format for the Situational Confidence Questionnaire. *Behav Res Ther.* **38**, 1211–1220.
10. Cherpitel, C.J. (1997) Brief screening instruments for alcoholism. *Alcohol Health Res World* **21**(4), 348–351.
11. Rollnick, S. *et al.* (1996) The development of a brief scale to measure outcome expectations of reduced consumption among excessive drinkers. *Addict Behav.* **21**(3), 377–387.
12. Samet, J.H. *et al.* (1996) Beyond CAGE: A brief clinical approach after detection of substance abuse. *Arch Internal Med.* **156**, 2287–2293.

13. Sklar, S.M. and Turner, N.E. (1999) A brief measure for the assessment of coping self-efficacy among alcohol and other drug users. *Addiction* **94**(5), 723–729.
14. Sobell, L.C. and Sobell, M.B. (1998) Identification and assessment of alcohol problems, in *Psychologist's Desk Reference* (eds G.P. Koocher *et al.*), Oxford University Press: New York, pp. 62–67.
15. Sobell, L.C. and Sobell, M.B. (2000) Drug abuse, in *Encyclopedia of Psychology* (ed. A.E. Kazdin), American Psychological Association and Oxford University Press: New York and Washington, DC, pp. 93–97.
16. Fleming, M. and Manwell, L.B. (1999) Brief intervention in primary care settings: A primary treatment method for at-risk, problem, and dependent drinkers. *Alcohol Health Res World* **23**(2), 128–137.
17. Fleming, M.F. *et al.* (1999) Brief physician advice for alcohol problems in older adults: A randomized community-based trial. *J Fam Pract.* **48** 378–384 (1999).
18. Heather, N. (1990) *Brief Intervention Strategies*, Pergamon: New York (Handbook of Alcoholism Treatment Approaches: Effective Alternatives).
19. Heather, N. (1994) Brief interventions on the world map. *Addiction* **89**, 665–667.
20. Rollnick, S. *et al.* (1997) Helping smokers make decisions: The enhancement of brief interventions for general medical practice. *Patient Educ Counseling* **31**, 191–203.
21. McLellan, A.T. *et al.* (1992) The fifth edition of the Addiction Severity Index. *J Subst Abuse Treatment* **9**, 199–213.
22. Allen, J.P. *et al.* (1997) A review of research on the Alcohol Use Disorders Identification Test (AUDIT). *Alcohol: Clin Experiment Res.* **21**, 613–619.
23. Saunders, J.B. *et al.* (1993) Development of the Alcohol Use Disorders Identification Test (AUDIT): Who collaborative project on early detection of persons with harmful alcohol consumption – II, *Addiction* **88**, 791–804.
24. Skinner, H.A. (1982) The Drug Abuse Screening Test. *Addict Behav* **7**, 363–371.
25. Rumpf, H.J. (1997) Development of a screening questionnaire for the general hospital and general practices. *Alcohol: Clin Exp Res.* **27**, 894–898.
26. Lesieur, H.R. and Blume, S.B. (1987) The South Oaks Gambling Screen in different settings. *J Gambling Stud.* **9**, 213–233.
27. Pomerleau, C.S. *et al.* (1990) Relationship between nicotine tolerance questionnaire scores and plasma cotinine *Addict Behav.* **15**, 73–80.
28. Fagerström, K.O. (1989) Measuring nicotine dependence: A review of the Fagerström Tolerance Questionnaire. *J Behav Med.* **12**, 159–182.
29. Sobell, L.C. *et al.* (1995) Reliability of a Drug History Questionnaire (DHQ). *Addict Behav.* **20**(2), 233–241.
30. Cyr, M.G. and Wartman, S.A. (1988) The effectiveness of routine screening questions in the detection of alcoholism. *J Am Med Assoc.* **259**, 51–54.
31. Taj, N. *et al.* Screening for problem drinking: Does a single question work? *J Fam Pract.* **46**, 328–335.
32. Woodruff, R.A. *et al.* (1976) A brief method of screening for alcoholism. *Dis Nerv Syst.* **37**, 434–435.
33. Korotitsch, W.J. and Nelson-Gray, R.O. (1999) An overview of self-monitoring research in assessment and treatment. *Psychol Assess.* **11** 415–425.
34. Marlatt, G.A. and Gordon, J.R. (1985) *Relapse Prevention*, Guilford Press: New York.
35. Annis, H.M. and Graham, J.M. (1988) *Situational Confidence Questionnaire (SCQ 39): User's Guide*, Addiction Research Foundation: Toronto.
36. May, R.K. *et al.* (1998) *The Situational Confidence Questionnaire for gambling: An initial psychometric evaluation*, Poster presented at the 32nd Annual Meeting of the Association for Advancement of Behavior Therapy November, 1998.
37. Sobell, L.C. *et al.* (1996) Fostering self-change among problem drinkers: A proactive community intervention. *Addict Behav.* **21**(6), 817–833.

38. Sobell, L.C. *et al.* (1993) What triggers the resolution of alcohol problems without treatment? *Alcohol: Clin Exp Res.* **17**(2) 217–224.
39. Sobell, M.B. and Sobell, L.C. (1998) Guiding self-change, in: *Treating Addictive Behaviors*, 2nd edn (eds W.R. Miller and N. Heather), Plenum: New York, pp. 189–202.
40. Cunningham, J.A. *et al.* (1993) Barriers to treatment: Why alcohol and drug abusers delay or never seek treatment. *Addict Behav.* **18**, 347–353.
41. Sobell, L.C. *et al.* (2000) Natural recovery from alcohol and drug problems: Methodological review of the research with suggestions for future directions. *Addiction* **95**, 749–769.
42. Sobell, L.C. *et al.* (eds) (1992) Recovery from alcohol problems without treatment, in *Self-Control and the Addictive Behaviors* (eds N. Heather, W.R. Miller and J. Greeley), Maxwell MacMillan: New York (Self-control and the addictive behaviours), pp. 198–242.
43. Miller, W.R. and Rollnick, S. (1991) *Motivational Interviewing: Preparing People to Change Addictive Behavior*, Guilford: New York.
44. Miller, W.R. and Tonigan, J.S. (1996) Assessing drinkers' motivation for change: The stages of change readiness and treatment eagerness scale (SOCRATES). *Psychol Addict Behav.* **10**(2), 81–89.